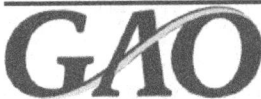

Report to the Chairman, Subcommittee on Livestock, Dairy, Poultry, Marketing and Agriculture Security, Committee on Agriculture, Nutrition and Forestry, U.S. Senate

August 2013

FOOD SAFETY

I0448880

More Disclosure and Data Needed to Clarify Impact of Changes to Poultry and Hog Inspections

August 2013

GAO Highlights

Highlights of GAO-13-775, a report to the Chairman, Subcommittee on Livestock, Dairy, Poultry, Marketing and Agriculture Security, Committee on Agriculture, Nutrition and Forestry, U.S. Senate

FOOD SAFETY

More Disclosure and Data Needed to Clarify Impact of Changes to Poultry and Hog Inspections

Why GAO Did This Study

USDA inspectors provide continuous inspection of each meat and poultry carcass and its parts that enter interstate commerce. In 1998, USDA began three pilot projects at slaughter plants for healthy young chickens, young turkeys, and young hogs, with a purpose to deploy inspection resources more effectively in accordance with food safety and other consumer protection requirements. Under the pilot projects, plant personnel sort carcasses before USDA's inspection. The pilot projects are to end when a final rule for each species is published. In January 2012, USDA published a proposed rule to modernize poultry slaughter inspections based, in part, on its pilot projects. GAO was asked to review these pilot projects. This report determines (1) the extent to which USDA has evaluated the three pilot projects, (2) strengths and weaknesses of the pilot projects based on the views of key stakeholder groups, and (3) the extent to which USDA disclosed limitations, if any, in sources of information it relied on to develop the proposed rule. GAO reviewed relevant laws and documents and interviewed USDA officials and 11 key industry, labor, consumer advocacy, and animal welfare groups familiar with the pilot projects.

What GAO Recommends

GAO recommends that USDA (1) collect and analyze information to determine if the young hog pilot project is meeting its purpose and (2) clearly disclose to the public limitations in the information it relied on for the proposed rule to modernize poultry slaughter inspections. USDA concurred with GAO's recommendations.

View GAO-13-775. For more information, contact J. Alfredo Gómez at (202) 512-3841 or gomezj@gao.gov.

What GAO Found

The U.S. Department of Agriculture (USDA) has not thoroughly evaluated the performance of each of the pilot projects over time even though the agency stated it would do so when it announced the pilot projects. For example, in 2011, USDA completed a report evaluating the pilot project at 20 young chicken plants concluding that an inspection system based on the pilot project would ensure equivalent, if not better, levels of food safety and quality than currently provided at plants not in the pilot project. However, among the limitations of its evaluation was the use of snapshots of data for two 2-year periods instead of data for the duration of the pilot project, which has been ongoing for more than a decade. In addition, USDA did not complete an evaluation on or prepare a report evaluating the pilot project at 5 young turkey plants and has no plans to do so because of the small sample size. Nevertheless, in publishing a proposed rule that includes an optional new poultry (chicken and turkey) inspection system, USDA stated that the new system was based on its experience with the pilot projects at young chicken and young turkey plants. As a result, USDA may not have assurance that its evaluation of the pilot project at young chicken plants provides the information necessary to support the proposed rule for both chickens and turkeys. However, the agency will not complete another evaluation before it issues a final rule. USDA has begun drafting a preliminary report evaluating the pilot project at young hog plants using analyses similar to those presented in the report evaluating young chicken plants, suggesting that similar limitations may apply. Agency officials stated that when USDA develops a proposed rulemaking to modify its slaughter inspection system for hogs, the agency will need to decide whether to collect additional data. Without collecting and analyzing additional data, it will be difficult for USDA to draw conclusions about whether the pilot project at young hog plants is meeting its purpose. While the pilot project is ongoing, USDA has the opportunity to collect and analyze additional information.

GAO identified strengths and weaknesses of the three pilot projects based on the views cited most frequently by 11 key stakeholder groups representing industry, labor, consumer advocacy, and animal welfare. On the basis of these views, GAO identified strengths including giving plants responsibility and flexibility for ensuring food safety and quality and allowing USDA inspectors to focus more on food safety activities. GAO identified weaknesses including that training of plant personnel assuming sorting responsibilities on the slaughter line is not required or standardized and that faster line speeds allowed under the pilot projects raise concerns about food safety and worker safety.

USDA did not disclose certain limitations in sources of information it relied on to develop the cost-benefit analysis supporting the proposed rule on modernizing poultry slaughter inspections. GAO identified three sources of information with certain limitations that were not disclosed. For example, USDA did not disclose that it gathered no cost information from young turkey plants in the pilot project. Furthermore, USDA generalized the results from 12 young chicken plants in the pilot project that responded to a 2001 cost survey to the universe of 335 young chicken and young turkey plants in the United States in 2012. As a result, stakeholders did not have complete and accurate information to inform their comments on the proposed rule and its potential impacts.

_____ **United States Government Accountability Office**

Contents

Abbreviations

CDC	Centers for Disease Control and Prevention
FSIS	Food Safety and Inspection Service
HACCP	Hazard Analysis and Critical Control Point
HIMP	HACCP-based Inspection Models Project
OMB	Office of Management and Budget
USDA	U.S. Department of Agriculture

GAO

U.S. GOVERNMENT ACCOUNTABILITY OFFICE

441 G St. N.W.
Washington, DC 20548

August 22, 2013

The Honorable Kirsten E. Gillibrand
Chairman
Subcommittee on Livestock, Dairy, Poultry, Marketing and Agriculture Security
Committee on Agriculture, Nutrition and Forestry
United States Senate

Dear Madam Chairman:

According to the Centers for Disease Control and Prevention (CDC), the U.S. food supply remains one of the safest in the world; nevertheless, CDC estimates that each year about 48 million Americans become sick from foodborne diseases. Meat and poultry products contaminated with pathogens such as *Salmonella, Toxoplasma gondii, Campylobacter*, and *Lysteria monocytogenes* cause many foodborne illnesses and deaths. To control the spread of such foodborne illnesses, over 3,700 U.S. Department of Agriculture (USDA) veterinarians and inspectors work at more than 900 slaughter plants. USDA inspectors provide continuous inspection of each meat and poultry carcass and its parts that enter interstate commerce. USDA inspectors positioned on slaughter lines in these plants are responsible for sorting carcasses to identify defects and directing plant personnel to remove unacceptable carcasses, among other things.[1] There may be multiple USDA inspectors positioned on each slaughter line, depending on the speed at which meat and poultry carcasses move down the line. For example, at plants that slaughter young chickens, there may be up to four inspectors on each line, and each inspector is responsible for inspecting up to 35 carcasses per minute. In addition, USDA inspectors positioned off the slaughter line move freely about the plant and collect samples of carcasses to test for microbial pathogens (e.g., *Salmonella*); perform food safety checks, such as verifying that carcasses are free of fecal material; and ensure that

---

[1]In slaughter plants that have received USDA approval to be inspected by USDA and thereby produce meat and poultry products to ship in interstate commerce (referred to as receiving a grant of inspection), there is a slaughter production line made up of multiple operations, beginning with the arrival of the animal in the receiving yard to the point where carcasses are chilled before they are further processed. In this report, we use the term "slaughter line" to refer to the entire slaughter production line that includes these multiple operations.

GAO-13-775 USDA Inspection Pilot Projects

carcasses comply with the agency's food quality standards for things such as bruises on chickens, which does not affect food safety.

In 1997, USDA announced the need to modify its meat and poultry slaughter inspection program to, among other things, make industry more responsible for identifying carcass defects. In 1998, USDA began three pilot projects—one for each species—at slaughter plants to test changes to its inspection systems from having its inspectors provide continuous inspection of each and every carcass for healthy young chickens, young turkeys, and young hogs to a system that uses plant personnel to examine each carcass for safety and quality and USDA inspectors to verify that safety and quality standards are met.[2] According to a *Federal Register* notice announcing the pilot projects, the purpose was to deploy inspection resources more effectively in accordance with food safety and other consumer protection requirements.[3] In announcing the pilot projects, USDA stated that the agency would thoroughly evaluate the pilot projects and, at the time of its evaluation, determine whether further testing should be conducted or whether to initiate rulemakings to adopt and implement new inspection systems based on the pilot projects. As of July 2013, 29 plants were participating in the pilot projects—19 plants for slaughtering young chickens, 5 for young turkeys, and 5 for young hogs. At participating plants under the pilot projects, plant personnel have taken on the sorting responsibilities of USDA inspectors positioned on the slaughter line for identifying carcass defects and removing unacceptable carcasses. However, a USDA inspector remains at the end of each slaughter line at each young chicken and young turkey plant and at three fixed locations on the slaughter line at each young hog plant to conduct a carcass-by-carcass inspection after plant personnel have completed sorting activities so that only those carcasses deemed likely to pass

---

[2]USDA refers to young hogs as market hogs.

[3]62 Fed. Reg. 31553 (June 10, 1997). Other consumer protection requirements include activities related to nonfood safety concerns, such as the wholesomeness and food quality of meat and poultry products. According to this *Federal Register* notice, USDA intended to test these changes at slaughter plants for young chickens, market hogs, and cattle. USDA extended the pilot projects to slaughter plants for young turkeys at the request of the turkey industry. According to USDA documents, no slaughter plants for young cattle have volunteered for the pilot project. Plants that slaughter young animals were selected because most food animals are slaughtered at a young age and because young animals are generally free of diseases that are more common in older animals.

inspection remain on the line.[4] According to a *Federal Register* notice, removing USDA inspectors from slaughter lines is intended to free the inspectors to perform additional food safety and quality checks in the areas of greatest risk, as needed, throughout the plant.

In December 2001, we reported on the design and methodology of USDA's pilot projects and noted several limitations that do not allow results from plants participating in USDA's pilot projects to be generalized to the universe of plants.[5] For example, we reported that plants participating in the young chicken pilot project were not randomly selected and that they did not include plants from all chicken producing areas or plants of all sizes. Thus, the results cannot be generalized to the entire population of chicken slaughter plants in the United States.

In January 2012, USDA published in the *Federal Register* a proposed rule to modernize poultry slaughter inspections that affects all plants that slaughter poultry (chickens and turkeys) and that includes an optional new inspection system for all young chicken and turkey plants, which resembles some aspects of the inspection systems used in the pilot projects at young chicken and young turkey plants.[6] During the public comment phase of the proposed rule for modernizing poultry slaughter inspections, USDA received more than 175,000 comments from stakeholders, including industry and consumer advocacy groups, as well as individual members of the public. As of July 2013, USDA was working to complete its final rule for modernizing poultry slaughter inspections, according to agency officials.

---

[4]USDA's original design for the pilot projects involved assigning inspectors to the slaughter line, but not at fixed points; instead these inspectors positioned off the line (i.e., not at a specific point on the line) could move freely to observe different parts of the line. However, in 1998, the union representing USDA inspectors filed a lawsuit claiming that, under the pilot projects, USDA inspectors were not complying with the applicable laws and personally inspecting each carcass. Consequently, in 2000, USDA modified the design of the pilot projects to include at least one USDA inspector positioned at a fixed point on the slaughter line to perform a carcass-by-carcass inspection. The court concluded that, with this modification, the pilot projects did not violate the applicable laws.

[5]GAO, *Food Safety: Weaknesses in Meat and Poultry Inspection Pilot Should Be Addressed before Implementation,* GAO-02-59 (Washington, D.C.: Dec. 17, 2001).

[6]77 Fed. Reg. 4408 (Jan. 27, 2012).

This report responds to your request that we review USDA's pilot projects at slaughter plants for young chickens, young turkeys, and young hogs. Our objectives were to determine (1) the extent to which USDA has evaluated the three pilot projects, (2) strengths and weaknesses of the three pilot projects based on the views of key stakeholder groups, and (3) the extent to which USDA disclosed limitations, if any, in sources of information it relied on to develop the proposed rule to modernize poultry slaughter inspections.

To determine the extent to which USDA has evaluated the three pilot projects, we reviewed relevant USDA documents, *Federal Register* notices, and laws. We also compared USDA's efforts to evaluate the pilot projects with criteria based on social science and evaluation literature and published GAO guidance identified in our previous work on pilot program development and evaluation.[7] In addition, we interviewed several officials in various offices within USDA's Food Safety and Inspection Service (FSIS)—the agency responsible for USDA's meat and poultry inspection program. To determine the strengths and weaknesses of the three pilot projects based on the views of key stakeholder groups, we identified 11 key stakeholder groups representing industry, labor (including plant personnel and USDA inspectors and veterinarians), consumer advocacy, and animal welfare with sufficient knowledge about USDA's three pilot projects that submitted comments on USDA's proposed rule on modernizing poultry slaughter inspections.[8] We reviewed their comments to determine the extent to which the comments may apply to the pilot

---

[7]GAO, *Catastrophic Planning: States Participating in FEMA's Pilot Program Made Progress, but Better Guidance Could Enhance Future Pilot Programs,* GAO-11-383 (Washington, D.C.: Apr. 8, 2011); GAO, *Tax Administration: IRS Needs to Strengthen Its Approach for Evaluating the SRFMI Data-Sharing Pilot Program,* GAO-09-45 (Washington, D.C.: Nov. 7, 2008); and GAO, *Equal Employment Opportunity: DOD's EEO Pilot Program Under Way, but Improvements Needed to DOD's Evaluation Plan,* GAO-06-538 (Washington, D.C.: May 5, 2006).

[8]We developed an initial list of key stakeholder groups based on our prior experience and knowledge. To ensure that we included all of the relevant stakeholder groups, we asked these groups for suggestions on other stakeholders we should consider contacting and expanded the list, as needed. The 11 stakeholder groups were the American Federation of Government Employees/National Joint Council of Food Inspection Locals, the American Meat Institute, the Center for Foodborne Illness Research and Prevention, the Consumer Federation of America, Food and Water Watch, the Government Accountability Project, the Humane Society of the United States, the National Association of Federal Veterinarians, the National Chicken Council, the National Turkey Federation, and the North American Meat Association.

projects; interviewed representatives of these key stakeholder groups; and followed up with e-mailed questions to gauge their level of familiarity with each pilot project and then clarified responses, as needed. We developed categories of strengths and weaknesses identified most frequently by stakeholder groups and determined whether each stakeholder group had identified strengths or weaknesses that fit into these categories. To determine the extent to which USDA disclosed limitations, if any, in sources of information it relied on to develop the proposed rule, we reviewed the proposed rule and related *Federal Register* notices, as well as selected documents the agency relied on to develop the proposed rule. We also interviewed several officials in various offices within USDA's FSIS to clarify information, as needed. Appendix I provides more information on our objectives, scope, and methodology.

We conducted this performance audit from September 2012 to August 2013 in accordance with generally accepted government auditing standards. Those standards require that we plan and perform the audit to obtain sufficient, appropriate evidence to provide a reasonable basis for our findings and conclusions based on our audit objectives. We believe that the evidence presented provides a reasonable basis for our findings and conclusions based on our audit objectives.

Background

The Federal Meat Inspection Act and the Poultry Products Inspection Act give USDA overall responsibility for ensuring the safety and wholesomeness of meat and poultry products that enter interstate commerce.[9] Acting under these legislative authorities, USDA inspectors provide continuous government inspection of each and every meat and poultry carcass and its parts at slaughter plants throughout the United States. Within USDA, FSIS is responsible for inspections at all meat and poultry slaughter and processing plants and has inspectors positioned both on and off the slaughter line. FSIS inspectors positioned on the line are to inspect every carcass and its parts, including the viscera (e.g., hearts and liver) organoleptically—by sight, touch, and smell—for defects, and direct plant personnel to take appropriate corrective action when

---

[9]21 U.S.C. §§ 601-683 and 21 U.S.C. 451-472. The Federal Meat Inspection Act was originally enacted in 1907 as part of the USDA appropriations act, and the Poultry Products Inspection Act was enacted in 1957. Both pieces of legislation have been amended a number of time throughout the years.

defects are found. According to a *Federal Register* notice, plants rely on FSIS inspectors to control and direct their production processes. For example, FSIS regulates the speed of the slaughter line based on its inspectors' ability to perform proper inspection procedures. FSIS inspectors positioned off the line move freely about the plant to focus on areas of greatest risk and to perform collection of carcass samples for testing of microbial pathogens. Among other activities, these inspectors review plant records and live animals presented for slaughter. These inspectors are also responsible for ensuring plants' compliance with regulatory requirements on a daily basis and for taking regulatory enforcement action when deficiencies are found.

In 1997, FSIS announced the need to modify its meat and poultry slaughter inspection program to, among other things, make industry more responsible for identifying carcass defects. This approach is consistent with the agency's previous adoption of the Pathogen Reduction: Hazard Analysis and Critical Control Point (HACCP) regulations. Under the risk-based HACCP approach, industry—rather than federal inspectors—is responsible for identifying steps in food production where food safety hazards, such as fecal material, are reasonably likely to occur and for establishing controls that prevent or reduce these hazards. As part of this approach, plants must identify the point (known as the critical control point) where they will establish control for a food safety hazard and take steps to prevent, eliminate, or control the hazard. FSIS had not extended the HACCP principles to slaughter inspections because the agency provides continuous inspection of each and every carcass. However, FSIS believed that changing its existing inspection systems would also reduce inspectors' reliance on organoleptic inspections, allow for a shift to prevention-oriented inspection systems based on risk, and permit redeployment of its resources to better protect the public from foodborne diseases. Before making a permanent change to its slaughter inspection systems, FSIS developed the pilot projects in 1998 at young chicken, young turkey, and young hog plants to test whether such a change would achieve its intended purpose of deploying inspection resources more effectively in accordance with food safety and other consumer protection requirements. FSIS' pilot projects at these plants are known as the HACCP-based Inspection Models Project (HIMP).

FSIS developed food safety and quality performance standards for plants in the pilot projects to meet.[10] FSIS set the performance standard for food safety defects at zero.[11] An example of a food safety defect is a carcass contaminated with fecal material because ingestion of meat and poultry contaminated with fecal material poses potential harm to humans. FSIS' performance standards for food quality defects vary, depending on the animal species and the type of defects. An example of a food quality defect is bruises on the carcass that, while not harmful if consumed, affects the wholesomeness of meat and poultry products. According to FSIS officials, the food quality performance standards are intended to be more stringent than the performance standards in place at plants that are not participating in the pilot projects.

In May 1999, FSIS negotiated an agreement with the union representing its inspectors that limited the number of plants participating in the pilot projects to 20 young chicken plants, 5 young turkey plants, and 5 young hog plants. According to the agreement, the pilot projects for each species are to end when a final rule is published for that species. Before converting to the inspection systems under the pilot projects, participating plants modified their operations to meet certain requirements, such as installing a new workstation at the end of the slaughter line and before the chiller for the FSIS inspector positioned on the slaughter line at poultry plants.[12] Over the course of the pilot projects, some plants have dropped out, and others have joined. As of July 2013, 29 plants were participating in the pilot projects in 18 states. Appendix II provides additional information on the location of plants in the pilot projects and the volume of poultry and hog slaughter in the United States.

In 2006, FSIS announced a voluntary initiative—known as the Salmonella Initiative Program—to make improvements to control for *Salmonella* at

---

[10]FSIS took a statistically based number of samples to develop these performance standards. In 2002, an external review concluded that the agency's approach for comparing food safety and quality data to assess the performance of chicken plants in the pilot project against the performance standards was valid.

[11]The agency has a performance standard of zero for food safety defects (i.e., septicemia/toxemia and visible fecal material) in plants participating and not participating in the pilot projects.

[12]The chiller is the point when eviscerated carcasses—carcasses that have had internal organs and any processing defects removed—are chilled in order to inhibit microbial growth and meet the regulatory requirements of 9 C.F.R. § 381.66(b)(1).

young chicken and turkey plants. Plants participating in FSIS' pilot projects are required to participate in this program. The Salmonella Initiative Program permits plants to operate with an exemption (known as a waiver) from complying with certain regulatory requirements. For example, young chicken plants in the pilot project are exempt from meeting FSIS' regulatory requirement that limits the slaughter line speed at young chicken plants and can operate the slaughter line at a faster line speed. Plants in the Salmonella Initiative Program must demonstrate to FSIS that results from their *Salmonella* testing consistently demonstrate that they maintain control over production processes. The goal of the Salmonella Initiative Program is to reduce and eliminate *Salmonella* before products reach consumers.

In January 2012, FSIS published in the *Federal Register* a proposed rule to modernize poultry slaughter inspections based, in part, on the agency's experience with the pilot projects at young chicken and young turkey plants. FSIS developed the proposed rule in response to an executive order directing agencies to review existing regulations that may have been outdated and modify them accordingly.[13] According to the proposed rule, the modernization is intended to improve food safety and the effectiveness of poultry slaughter inspection systems, remove unnecessary regulatory obstacles to innovation, and make better use of the agency's resources. The proposed rule further states that inspection systems currently in place at chicken and turkey plants (not in the pilot projects) are lacking in two important respects. First, the proper role of industry and FSIS is obscured. Specifically, FSIS inspectors are currently responsible for sorting acceptable carcasses from unacceptable carcasses, finding defects, identifying corrective actions, and solving problems in production control processes, but these are roles more appropriately the responsibility of the slaughter plants. Second, a significant amount of FSIS' inspection program personnel resources are allocated toward inspection activities to detect defects and conditions that present minimal food safety risks. According to the proposed rule, this allocation limits the agency resources available for food safety-related inspection activities. Moreover, FSIS developed an economic cost and benefit analysis to demonstrate the merits of the proposed rule, which,

---

[13]As part of Executive Order 13563, federal agencies were asked to review existing rules that may be outmoded, ineffective, insufficient, or excessively burdensome and to modify, streamline, expand, or repeal them accordingly.

according to USDA, is expected to have an annual impact on the economy of more than $100 million.

FSIS' proposed rule affects all poultry slaughter plants and includes mandatory regulatory changes. For example, the proposed rule requires all poultry plants to maintain written procedures to prevent contamination of carcasses and parts by fecal material and pathogens (e.g., *Salmonella* and *Campylobacter*) and to test for organisms (e.g., *Salmonella*) to demonstrate control over their production processes at a point before the carcass enters the chiller and at a point after the carcass exits the chiller. In addition, the proposed rule includes the optional new poultry inspection system for young chicken and turkey plants.[14] According to the proposed rule, FSIS expects that the majority of young chicken and turkey plants will convert to the optional new poultry inspection system. The new poultry inspection system resembles the inspection systems at young chicken and young turkey plants in the pilot projects but also has some differences. Similarities between the pilot projects and optional new poultry inspection system include, among others:

- For each slaughter line, there would be one FSIS inspector positioned at the end of the line to perform a carcass-by-carcass inspection and one FSIS inspector positioned off the line to perform, among other things, food safety and quality checks on carcasses to verify that plant personnel (known as sorters) have effectively performed their duties, such as removing fecal material on carcasses.
- The FSIS inspector positioned on the slaughter line would visually inspect (observe) each carcass after the viscera are separated from it and after plant personnel have sorted carcasses, at a point near the end of the slaughter line.

A difference between the pilot projects and the optional new poultry inspection system is that the new system would eliminate FSIS' performance standards for food quality defects and replace them with a requirement that plants maintain records documenting that their products meet the regulatory definition of "ready-to-cook." Ready-to-cook means that the products are free of such defects as feathers, oil glands, and

---

[14]The proposed rule will also include updates to the traditional inspection system typically in place at smaller, lower volume producing plants that eviscerate carcasses by hand. According to the proposed rule, a plant can choose to operate under the optional new poultry inspection system or the updated traditional inspection system.

diseases and are thus suitable for cooking without any further preparation. According to FSIS officials, plants could use the existing food quality standards—known as Finished Product Standards—to meet the regulatory definition of ready-to-cook.

FSIS Has Not Thoroughly Evaluated the Three Pilot Projects

FSIS has not thoroughly evaluated the performance of each of the three pilot projects over time even though the agency stated that it would do so when it announced the pilot projects. Specifically, FSIS completed a report evaluating the pilot project at young chicken plants, but its data analyses have limitations. FSIS did not prepare a report evaluating the pilot project at young turkey plants and has no plans to do so because data from the five young turkey plants in the pilot project provide limited information due to the small sample size. While FSIS has begun drafting a preliminary report evaluating the pilot project at young hog plants, it used analyses similar to those presented in the report evaluating the pilot project at young chicken plants, suggesting similar limitations may apply.

FSIS Has Completed a Report Evaluating Some Data from the Chicken Pilot Project, but Its Data Analyses Have Limitations

In 2011, FSIS completed a report evaluating the pilot project at young chicken plants;[15] according to agency officials, the agency's evaluation efforts focused on this pilot project, in part, because it has the largest number of plants participating. FSIS' evaluation compared the performance of the 20 young chicken plants in the pilot project (1) with a similar group of 64 plants not participating in the pilot project,[16] using routinely collected data, and (2) against the performance standards developed for the pilot project using data collected specifically for the pilot project. FSIS' evaluation concludes that an inspection system based on the pilot project would ensure equivalent, if not better, levels of food safety and quality than currently provided at plants not in the pilot project. FSIS used this evaluation to support its January 2012 proposed rule modernizing poultry slaughter inspections that includes the optional new poultry inspection system.

---

[15]USDA, Food Safety and Inspection Service, *Evaluation of HACCP Inspection Models Project (HIMP)*, August 2011. FSIS' evaluation included 20 young chicken plants participating in the pilot project; however, one plant dropped out of the pilot project in 2011 and closed its operations after the evaluation had been completed.

[16]For the similar group of plants, FSIS selected plants that had similar slaughter volumes and line speeds and that were located in similar geographic areas in the United States.

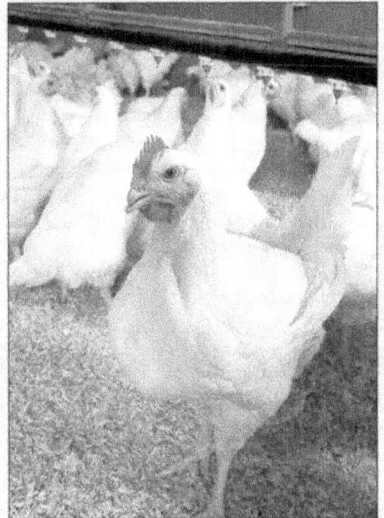
We identified two limitations of FSIS' evaluation that raise questions about the validity of FSIS' conclusion that an inspection system based on the pilot project would ensure equivalent, if not better, levels of food safety and quality than currently provided at plants not in the pilot project. First, FSIS' conclusion about the pilot project was based, in part, on comparisons of data that were not designed to be comparable. For example, FSIS concluded that the prevalence of *Salmonella* at the 20 plants participating in the pilot project was significantly lower than in the similar group of 64 plants that were not participating in the pilot project from 2006 to 2008. However, it based its conclusion on data that were collected as a part of its microbial sampling program, rather than collecting samples from the same plants for each year. The total number of samples collected in each year declined from one year to the next— indicating that the total number of plants from which samples was collected varied from year to year (see fig. 1).[17] FSIS officials confirmed that the total number of plants from which samples were collected varied from year to year, and these officials were unable to tell us how many plants were included in each year of the analysis. In addition, the possibility that lower prevalence of *Salmonella* was caused by something other than the pilot project cannot be ruled out.

---

[17]FSIS' performance standards call for a series of samples be collected over 51 consecutive days at each plant selected to be part of the annual sampling schedule. Plants included in the annual schedule are selected on risk-based criteria designed to focus FSIS resources on plants with the most samples positive for *Salmonella*.

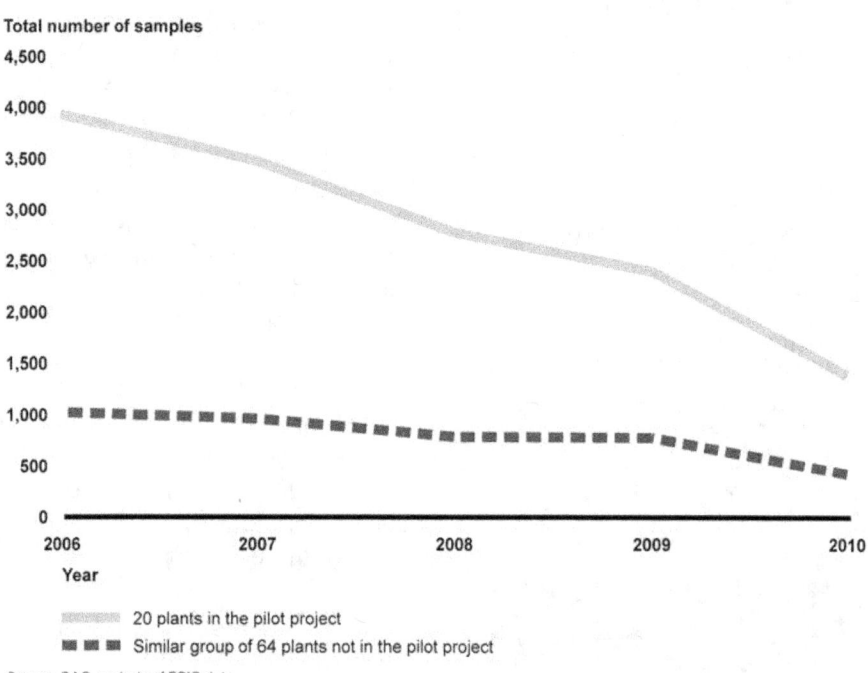

Figure 1: Total Number of Samples Collected at the 20 Young Chicken Plants in the Pilot Project and the Similar Group of 64 Young Chicken Plants Not in the Pilot Project, 2006-2010

Total number of samples

20 plants in the pilot project

Similar group of 64 plants not in the pilot project

Source: GAO analysis of FSIS data.

Moreover, data from the last 2 years analyzed did not show a significantly lower prevalence of *Salmonella* for plants participating in the pilot project. According to FSIS officials, FSIS did not collect data to demonstrate the relative effectiveness of plants participating and not participating in any of the pilot projects. Instead, the agency analyzed data for a variety of inspection activities performed in all plants (regardless of a plant's inspection system) to ensure their compliance with regulatory requirements.

The second limitation that we identified in FSIS' evaluation is that the agency collected more than a decade's worth of data on the extent to which young chicken plants in the pilot project were meeting the food safety and quality performance standards developed for the pilot project, but it based its conclusion about the performance of the pilot project on the use of snapshots of data from the pilot project for two 2-year periods. Moreover, the time frames for the snapshots differed depending on whether the categories related to food safety or food quality defects. More specifically, the agency included snapshots of food safety data from 2000 to 2002—when the project first began—and food safety data from April 2009 to March 2011, and snapshots of food quality data from 2000 to 2002 with food quality data from 2009 to 2010—the most recent data available at that time. Consequently, the results from the years that FSIS selected for analysis may not be indicative of plants' performance over time. According to FSIS officials, the agency did not analyze the data for the majority of the years because the data were recorded on paper forms stored at individual plants and compiling the data for analysis was labor intensive.[18] According to the *Standards for Internal Control in the Federal Government*,[19] federal agencies are to employ internal control activities, such as top-level review, to help ensure that management's directives are carried out and to determine if agencies are effectively and efficiently using resources. Without analyzing data for the majority of the years of the pilot project in its evaluation, FSIS could not determine whether an inspection system based on the pilot project would ensure equivalent, if not better, levels of food safety and quality than currently provided at plants not in the pilot project over time. In addition, according to the *Federal Register* notice announcing the pilot projects, FSIS stated that the agency would thoroughly evaluate them; however, using snapshots of data rather than data for the majority of the years of the pilot project, the agency did not conduct a thorough evaluation. Instead, FSIS veterinarians and inspectors evaluated the performance of their individual plants against regulatory performance standards on a daily basis, as they routinely do for all plants regardless of whether they are in the pilot project or not, as well as the performance standards for the pilot project. However, the agency has not aggregated and analyzed these daily results to determine how the plants participating in the pilot project have performed over time.

Notwithstanding these limitations, FSIS used its evaluation of the pilot project at young chicken plants to support the proposed rule on modernizing poultry slaughter inspections. Moreover, the design and methodology limitations we identified in our 2001 report (e.g., young chicken plants participating in the pilot project constituted a small,

---

[18]FSIS has been collecting similar data in a similar format at the young turkey and young hog plants participating in the pilot projects.

[19]GAO, *Standards for Internal Control in the Federal Government*, GAO/AIMD-00-21.3.1 (Washington, D.C.: Nov. 1999).

nonrandom sample) continue to prevent the results obtained from the 20 participating young chicken plants from being generalized to the 239 young chicken plants and 96 young turkey plants in the United States in 2012. As a result, FSIS may not have assurance that its evaluation of the pilot project at young chicken plants provides the information necessary to support the proposed rule for poultry—both chickens and turkeys. However, according to the *Federal Register* notice supporting the proposed rule on modernizing poultry slaughter inspections, the agency conducted a comprehensive evaluation; thus, the agency will not complete another evaluation before it issues a final rule.

FSIS Did Not Prepare a Report Evaluating the Turkey Pilot Project

Unlike what FSIS did for the pilot project at young chicken plants, it did not complete an evaluation on or prepare a report evaluating the pilot project at young turkey plants. In publishing the proposed rule modernizing poultry slaughter inspections that included an optional new poultry inspection system, the agency stated that the new system was based on its experience with the pilot projects at young chicken and young turkey plants. According to FSIS officials, the agency did not prepare a report evaluating the pilot project at young turkey plants and has no plans to do so because data from five young turkey plants in the pilot project provide limited information due to the small sample size.

Instead, as part of a quantitative microbial risk assessment to estimate the public health impact of the proposed rule, the agency analyzed the relationship between the presence or absence of pathogens and the frequency with which FSIS inspectors positioned off the slaughter line carried out specific inspection activities at young turkey plants.[20] According to FSIS' analysis, there is a suggested relationship between young turkey plants' participation in the pilot project and a lower prevalence of *Salmonella* and *Campylobacter*.

In addition, FSIS officials stated that, for the optional new poultry inspection system, they generalized information and data from young chicken plants in the pilot project to the young turkey plants in the pilot project because the processes to slaughter chickens and turkeys are

Turkey Production, Slaughter, and Export

The United States is the world's largest turkey producer, followed by the European Union, according to the U.S. Department of Agriculture (USDA). In 2012, about 249 million young turkeys were slaughtered at 96 plants, primarily in the Midwestern and Eastern United States. According to the National Turkey Federation, Americans consumed about 16 pounds of turkey per person in 2011. Also, most turkey companies are vertically integrated, meaning they control or contract for all phases of production and processing. According to USDA, in 2012, the United States exported 800 million pounds of turkey meat, over half of which was destined for Mexico, and about 167 million pounds of turkey viscera (e.g., heart and liver), with the largest amount (about 45 million pounds) going to China (including Hong Kong).

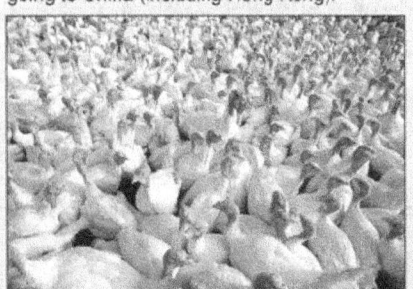

Source: USDA.

[20]USDA/FSIS, *FSIS Risk Assessment for Guiding Public Health-Based Poultry Slaughter Inspection,* Updated November 2011. In this assessment, FSIS evaluated inspection data and *Salmonella* and *Campylobacter* data from young turkey slaughter plants as a part of its peer reviewed risk assessment.

similar. However, we identified differences in the food quality performance standards and FSIS' testing protocol for pathogens. FSIS acknowledged that the food quality performance standards are not the same. We determined that the five food quality performance standards developed for the young chicken and for the young turkey pilot project can differ by 0.5 percent to almost 16 percent. For example, the performance standard for the food quality defect category that includes animal diseases (such as arthritis) is 1.7 percent for young chickens and 1.2 percent for young turkeys—a difference of 0.5 percent. In another example, the performance standard for the food quality defect that includes other defects such as feathers is 80.0 percent for young chickens and 95.9 percent for young turkeys—a difference of 15.9 percent.

Furthermore, FSIS' protocols differ for testing chicken and turkey carcasses for *Salmonella* and *Campylobacter*. For example, for chickens, FSIS inspectors rinse an entire chicken carcass in a bag filled with a sterile water solution that is poured off and tested for these pathogens. In contrast, for turkeys, FSIS inspectors use a sponge—containing the same sterile water solution as that used to rinse chicken carcasses—to swab certain areas of the turkey carcass and then test the sponge for pathogens. According to a March 2011 *Federal Register* notice,[21] FSIS acknowledged that the method used to sample carcasses affects the results and stated that they are not proposing to compare microbial data from these two species. However, even with these differences in sampling protocols, FSIS officials stated that the results for young chickens could be generalized to young turkeys. These differences raise questions about the extent to which FSIS can generalize results for food quality defects and microbial testing results from one species to the other, but, as we previously mentioned, the agency has no plans to do an evaluation of the pilot project at young turkey plants before it issues a final rule.

FSIS Has Not Completed Its Report Evaluating the Hog Pilot Project

In 2011, FSIS began drafting a preliminary report evaluating the pilot project at young hog plants. The preliminary report uses analyses similar to those presented in the report evaluating the pilot project at young chicken plants, suggesting that similar limitations may apply. In particular, FSIS did not collect comparable data from plants participating and not

---

[21]76 Fed. Reg. 15,282 (Mar. 21, 2011).

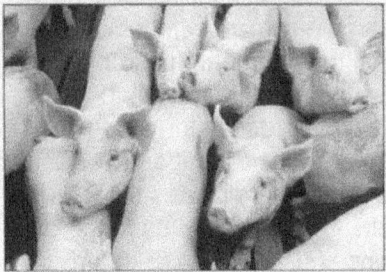
participating in the pilot project. In addition, like the turkey pilot project, information collected from the five young hog plants in the pilot project would not provide reasonable assurance that any conclusions can apply more broadly to the universe of 608 hog plants in the United States in 2012 because of the small sample size. FSIS officials agreed that there would be concerns regarding the strength of any conclusions based on five plants. These officials stated that, when the agency develops a proposed rulemaking to modify its slaughter inspection system for hogs, it will need to decide whether to collect additional data. Furthermore, a May 2013 USDA Office of Inspector General report identified areas of risk in FSIS' inspection of hog plants, including those participating in the pilot project.[22] The report found that FSIS did not critically assess whether the pilot project had measurably improved food safety at each participating plant because the agency did not adequately oversee the program.[23] In response, FSIS stated that it would complete an evaluation that would include an analysis of plants participating and not participating in the pilot project. However, as we previously stated, the analyses that the agency plans to use in this evaluation are similar to those presented in the report evaluating the pilot project at young chicken plants, suggesting that similar limitations may apply. According to FSIS officials, the agency intends to complete this evaluation by March 31, 2014. The officials said that the agency could use its final report evaluating the pilot project at young hog plants to support a rulemaking but currently has no time frame for doing so. FSIS' pilot project at young hog plants will end when a final rule for hog slaughter is published.

As FSIS officials stated, when the agency develops a proposed rulemaking to modify its slaughter inspection system for hogs, it will need to decide whether to collect additional data. However, while the pilot project is ongoing, FSIS has the opportunity to follow sound management practices by planning for and collecting key information needed to

---

[22]USDA, Office of Inspector General, *Food Safety and Inspection Service—Inspection and Enforcement Activities at Swine Slaughter Plants,* Audit Report 24601-0001-41, May 9, 2013.

[23]Although the pilot project was intended to improve food safety, the Office of Inspector General report found that 3 of the 10 plants cited with the most noncompliance with regulations from fiscal years 2008 to 2011 were plants in the pilot project. In fact, the hog plant with the most noncompliance during this time frame was a plant in the pilot project—with nearly 50 percent more noncompliance citations than the plant with the next highest number.

determine whether the pilot project is meeting its purpose. We have previously reported that pilot programs can more effectively inform future program rollout when sound management practices are followed.[24] Consistent with best practices in program management,[25] our guide for designing evaluations,[26] and our prior work, we identified sound management practices to design a pilot to guide consistent implementation, including the type and source of data needed to evaluate the pilot, and to conduct analysis of the results.

However, FSIS has not collected key information needed to determine whether the pilot project is meeting its purpose of deploying inspection resources more effectively in accordance with food safety and other consumer protection requirements. For example, FSIS has not collected information on the total costs of the pilot project to the agency or on any changes in the number of FSIS inspectors at the plants participating in the pilot project. Thus far, at young hog plants, FSIS veterinarians and inspectors have evaluated the performance of their individual plants against regulatory performance standards on a daily basis, as they routinely do for all plants regardless of whether they are in the pilot project or not, as well as the performance standards for the pilot project. However, the agency has not aggregated and analyzed these daily results to determine how the plants participating in the pilot project have performed over time. Without collecting and analyzing additional data, it

---

[24]See GAO-11-383, GAO-09-45, and GAO-06-538. Specifically, in GAO-11-383, GAO-09-45, and GAO-06-538, we reported that a sound, well-developed and documented evaluation plan includes, at a minimum: (1) well-defined, clear, and measurable objectives; (2) criteria or standards for determining pilot-program performance; (3) clearly articulated methodology, including sound sampling methods, determination of appropriate sample size for the evaluation design, and a strategy for comparing the pilot results with other efforts; (4) a clear plan that details the type and source of data necessary to evaluate the pilot, methods for data collection, and the timing and frequency of data collection; and (5) a data analysis plan to track the program's performance and evaluate the final results of the project.

[25]See, for example, P.H. Rossi, M.W. Lipsey, and H.E. Freeman, *Evaluation: A Systematic Approach* (Thousand Oaks, Calif.: 2004); and the Project Management Institute. *The Standard for Program Management®* (Newton Square, Pa.: 2006). Specifically, *Evaluation: A Systematic Approach* covers evaluation research activities used in appraising the design, implementation, effectiveness, and efficiency of social programs. Also, *The Standard for Program Management* describes program phases to facilitate program governance, enhanced control, and coordination of program and project resources and overall risk management.

[26]See, GAO, *Designing Evaluations*, GAO/PEMD-10.1.4 (Washington, D.C.: March 1991).

will be difficult for FSIS to draw conclusions about whether the pilot project at young hog plants is meeting its purpose of deploying inspection resources more effectively in accordance with food safety and other consumer protection requirements.

Views of Key Stakeholder Groups on Strengths and Weaknesses in the Pilot Projects

We identified strengths and weaknesses of the three pilot projects based on the views of 11 key stakeholder groups representing industry, labor, consumer advocacy, and animal welfare.[27] Strengths we identified in the pilot projects based on the views cited most frequently by stakeholder groups included the following:

- *Responsibility and flexibility.* Representatives of 7 stakeholder groups stated that the pilot projects give plants responsibility and flexibility for ensuring food safety and quality. For example, representatives of 1 stakeholder group stated that, under the pilot projects, plants had greater flexibility to place plant personnel where they were skilled, while a representative of another stakeholder group stated that the pilot projects gave plants responsibility for producing safe food and allowed plants the latitude to incorporate new methods to ensure food safety.
- *More focus on food safety.* Representatives of 5 stakeholder groups stated that the pilot projects allow FSIS to focus more on food safety activities. For example, a representative of 1 stakeholder group stated that, in the pilot projects, FSIS inspectors focused on carcass and verification activities designed to reduce the incidence of foodborne pathogens.
- *Potential job creation and increased production.* Representatives of 3 stakeholder groups stated that the pilot projects may result in potential job creation and increased production at plants. For example, a representative of 1 stakeholder group stated some plants that joined the pilot projects hired new workers, purchased additional equipment, and expanded their facilities. A representative of another stakeholder group stated that the pilot projects allowed plants to increase line speeds to process and sell a larger quantity of products.

---

[27]Representatives from stakeholder groups stated that they were most familiar with the pilot project at young chicken plants and generally were not as familiar with the pilot projects at young turkey or young hog plants. However, representatives stated that their comments generally applied across the three pilot projects, which were all designed to have plant personnel assume the sorting responsibilities of FSIS inspectors positioned on the line for identifying carcass defects and removing unacceptable carcasses.

U.S. Poultry and Hog Inspection

U.S. Department of Agriculture (USDA) inspectors are responsible for ensuring the safety and wholesomeness of meat and poultry products that enter interstate commerce. Inspectors must pass a written test and have either a bachelor's degree in a related field or 1 year of job-related experience. Inspectors also receive classroom, as well as training on the slaughter line in, among other things, how to detect diseases, abnormalities, and contamination by sight, touch, and smell.

Currently, USDA regulations limit the maximum slaughter line speed based on the total number of inspectors on the line. However, according to USDA officials, slaughter lines typically do not operate at these maximum speeds because they can only do so under optimal conditions, determined by, among other things, the health of the birds and type of equipment. For plants in the pilot projects, USDA originally did not establish maximum line speeds. However, according to USDA officials, the agency later established a maximum line speed of 175 carcasses per minute for participating young chicken plants. USDA did so because it found that lines in these plants were capable of operating faster, but that a USDA inspector could not effectively inspect under such conditions. USDA did not establish a maximum line speed at participating young turkey and young hog plants because these plants did not significantly increase their line speeds.

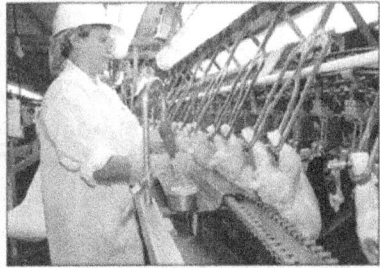

Source: USDA
In the above photo, a USDA inspector inspects young chicken carcasses separated from the viscera.

Weaknesses we identified in the pilot projects based on the views cited most frequently by stakeholder groups included the following:

- *Training*. Representatives from all 11 stakeholder groups stated that training for plant personnel that assume sorting responsibilities on the slaughter line is not required or standardized. For example, a representative of 1 stakeholder group stated that training of plant personnel was not required. Representatives of another stakeholder group stated that plants' training programs varied based on individual plant standards, and a representative of another stakeholder group recommended that FSIS provide detailed training and guidance on, among other things, conditions that require carcasses to be condemned to ensure that uniform standards are consistently used across industry in training plant personnel. According to FSIS officials, training of plant personnel was not required for plants participating in the pilot projects because, among other things, FSIS inspectors observed the line and made the plant take corrective actions, if necessary. Representatives of 3 stakeholder groups further noted that FSIS required that some countries, which exported to the United States and have similar inspection programs to the pilot projects, must train and certify their plant personnel. However, according to FSIS officials, the agency has no such requirement. Rather, FSIS officials stated that FSIS requires that foreign governments achieve an equivalent level of food safety protection as the U.S. inspection system, and that the countries, which stakeholders groups identified, chose to include training and certification requirements for their plant personnel to demonstrate this equivalence.
- *Line speed*. Representatives of 7 stakeholder groups stated that faster line speed creates food safety and worker safety concerns. For example, a representative of 1 stakeholder group stated that, at young chicken plants participating in the pilot project, the FSIS inspector on the line had about one second to inspect three carcasses, which was not enough time, especially if a bird was contaminated with a small amount of fecal material—posing a food safety concern. A representative of another stakeholder group stated that increased line speeds contributed to higher rates of carpal tunnel syndrome and other injuries in poultry plant personnel. According to FSIS' 2011 report evaluating the pilot project at young chicken plants, not all slaughter lines at the plants in the pilot project are running at their maximum speed. FSIS also noted in its report that young chicken plants operating under the pilot project demonstrated that they are capable of consistently producing safe poultry products and of consistently meeting pathogen reduction and other performance standards operating at these higher line speeds. However, as

previously noted in this report, we identified limitations in FSIS' evaluation. FSIS officials also told us that the agency is collaborating with the CDC's National Institute for Occupational Safety and Health to obtain data on the effects of increased line speed by collecting data at one young chicken plant, which is not participating in the pilot project, that has been granted a waiver from the line speed restriction under the Salmonella Initiative Program.[28]

- *Reduced ability to see potential defects.* Representatives of 5 stakeholder groups stated that FSIS inspectors' ability to see potential defects in young chicken carcasses is reduced because inspectors positioned on the slaughter line are observing the back of the carcass without the viscera. At young chicken plants not in the pilot project, FSIS inspectors examine the exterior, interior cavity, and viscera of each carcass. A representative of 1 stakeholder group noted that, at young chicken plants in the pilot project, inspectors positioned on the slaughter line can no longer see into the carcass' cavity, where fecal contamination was most likely to be located.[29] FSIS officials stated that inspectors observing the backs of chickens are able to identify fecal contamination, and they can require plant personnel to trim and reprocess contaminated carcasses. According to agency documents, observing the carcass without the viscera is sufficient for identifying all poultry diseases and conditions except for avian visceral leukosis, a viral disease that affects chickens. Because avian visceral leukosis is a condition that, if present, will be present throughout the entire flock, the agency has established a procedure at young chicken plants participating in the pilot project to observe the viscera of the first 300 birds of a flock near the beginning of the slaughter line to determine the presence of this condition.

- *Noncompliance with zero-tolerance standard for fecal material more difficult to cite.* Representatives of 5 stakeholder groups stated that it is harder for FSIS inspectors to cite plants for not complying with FSIS' zero-tolerance standard for fecal material because plants in the

---

[28]According to the CDC's website, the mission of the National Institute for Occupational Safety and Health is to generate new knowledge in the field of occupational safety and health and to transfer that knowledge into practice for the betterment of workers by conducting scientific research, developing guidance and authoritative recommendations, disseminating information, and responding to requests for workplace health hazard evaluations.

[29]In young chicken plants participating in the pilot project, inspectors view the backs of the carcasses after the birds have been sorted and cleaned and generally do not touch the carcasses.

pilot projects may decide to address a food safety hazard—such as fecal material—at a point on the slaughter line after the FSIS inspector.[30] For example, a representative of 1 stakeholder group raised a concern that by allowing plants in the pilot project to move the critical control point for preventing, eliminating, and controlling fecal material to a location on the slaughter line after the FSIS inspector, the FSIS inspector no longer had the ability to ensure that the plant complied with the standard to control for that hazard.[31] More specifically, the FSIS inspector positioned on the line could no longer cite the plant for noncompliance with FSIS' zero-tolerance standard for fecal material because the plant would not yet have had an opportunity to control for this hazard. In response, FSIS officials stated that there were more opportunities for identifying noncompliance with fecal standards for young poultry plants in the pilot projects because FSIS inspectors positioned off the slaughter line perform more food safety activities than at plants not participating in the pilot projects.

- *Conflict of interest of plant personnel sorting carcasses.* Representatives from 4 stakeholder groups stated that plants' responsibility for sorting carcasses presents a conflict of interest. For example, a representative of 1 stakeholder group expressed concern that a plant's financial incentive to process the maximum number of birds conflicted with its responsibility to regulate itself and stated that if plant personnel continually removed birds from the line, those personnel might be taken off the line. FSIS officials stated that plants' responsibility for sorting carcasses did not present a conflict of interest because FSIS inspectors performed food safety activities, inspected each carcass, and verified the effectiveness of plant personnel's sorting activities.

---

[30]At plants not participating in the pilot projects, FSIS inspectors positioned on the slaughter line sort carcasses and direct plant personnel to reprocess (remove) visible fecal material from the carcasses. These FSIS inspectors positioned on the slaughter line do not cite the plants for noncompliance with FSIS' zero-tolerance standard for fecal material.

[31]As previously stated, under the risk-based HACCP approach, plants must identify the point where they will control for food safety hazards, such as fecal material. Young chicken plants in the pilot project have discretion to establish the critical control point at a fixed location on the slaughter line either before or after the FSIS inspector's position on the slaughter line. If the critical control point is located before the FSIS inspector, then the inspector can cite the plant if the hazard is found. In contrast, if the critical control point is located after the FSIS inspector, then the inspector cannot cite the plant if the hazard is found.

- *Insufficient evidence of success of the pilot projects.* Representatives of 3 stakeholder groups stated that FSIS does not have sufficient evidence to demonstrate the success of the pilot projects. For example, a representative of 1 stakeholder group stated that FSIS' data from the pilot project at young chicken plants demonstrated that FSIS inspectors on the slaughter lines missed food safety defects on carcasses, such as fecal material. In particular, the stakeholder group representative cited FSIS data showing that FSIS inspectors positioned off the slaughter line who are responsible for, among other things, verifying the food safety of a sample of carcasses, found food safety defects at a much higher rate than FSIS inspectors positioned on the slaughter line. According to FSIS officials, the rate at which FSIS inspectors positioned on the slaughter line detected food safety defects was not directly comparable to the rate at which FSIS inspectors positioned off the slaughter line detected food safety defects because the inspectors positioned on the line and off the line had different but complementary roles. FSIS officials maintained, in its 2011 report evaluating the pilot project at young chicken plants, that the pilot project improved the safety of chicken products at participating plants. However, as previously noted in this report, we identified limitations in FSIS' evaluation.
- *Increased costs to industry.* Representatives of 2 stakeholder groups stated that the pilot projects can result in increased costs to industry for additional capital investment, training, and staff. For example, a representative of 1 stakeholder group stated that plants participating in the pilot projects may need substantial capital for redesigning equipment and adding personnel, and a representative of another stakeholder group noted that plants participating in the pilot projects needed to add plant personnel to replace FSIS inspectors. FSIS officials stated that participation in the pilot projects was voluntary and that plants could choose whether to invest capital when participating.

FSIS officials stated that they recognized there were similarities between the pilot projects and the optional new poultry inspection system included in the proposed rule, and they are working to address concerns identified by stakeholder groups in the final rule on modernizing poultry slaughter inspections.

FSIS Did Not Disclose Certain Limitations in the Cost-Benefit Analysis It Developed to Support the Proposed Rule

FSIS did not disclose certain limitations in sources of information it relied on to develop the cost-benefit analysis supporting the proposed rule on modernizing poultry slaughter inspections. As a result, the public, including stakeholders, did not have complete and accurate information to inform their comments on the proposed rule, including the uncertainty behind selected estimates. According to the Office of Management and Budget (OMB) Circular A-4,[32] which provides guidance to federal agencies on the development of regulatory analysis, and USDA's departmental regulation that details the process for developing regulations,[33] a good cost-benefit analysis is transparent and a qualified third party reading the analysis should be able to understand the basic elements.

We identified three sources of information FSIS used that contained certain limitations that were not disclosed in the cost-benefit analysis. First, in the 2012 proposed rule, FSIS did not disclose that it used a 2001 survey of plants' costs of converting to the pilot projects to estimate certain costs for a plant that slaughters young chickens or turkeys to operate under the optional new poultry inspection system. According to USDA's departmental regulation, the quality of the data used in cost-benefit analyses should be discussed in the proposed rule. However, our review of the proposed rule found the following limitations in the survey data that FSIS did not disclose:

- Estimated costs included in the January 2012 proposed rule were based on cost information gathered in 2001. FSIS officials told us that they did not attempt to obtain more recent information because it was challenging to collect this type of information from plants, which consider such information proprietary. FSIS officials stated that there has been little or no change in the cost information but did not provide any documentation to support this statement.
- FSIS generalized the results from the 12 young chicken plants that responded to the 2001 cost survey to the universe of 335 young chicken and young turkey plants in the United States in 2012 to estimate certain costs for poultry plants to operate under the optional new poultry inspection system. However, results obtained from the 12

---

[32]OMB, Circular A-4, Sept. 17, 2003.

[33]USDA, Departmental Regulation, No. 1512, Regulatory Decision Making Requirements, Dec. 24, 2008.

young chicken plants that responded to the survey are not representative of the universe of young poultry plants.

- For the young turkey plants participating in the pilot project, FSIS did not obtain any cost data. According to FSIS officials, the agency did not attempt to obtain cost information from participating young turkey plants because, at the time of the 2001 survey, there were only two such plants. These officials further stated that the process to slaughter chickens is sufficiently similar to that for turkeys so costs can be generalized. However, these officials acknowledged there are differences between chickens and turkeys, such as carcass size, that can affect costs, including chilling costs.

As a result of these limitations, the costs for a plant to convert to the optional new poultry inspection system in today's economy may be unclear to the public, including stakeholders.

Second, to estimate selected benefits of the proposed rule, FSIS assumed a single value for certain economic parameters, rather than following USDA's departmental regulation and OMB's Circular A-4 and using a sensitivity analysis to provide for a range of uncertainty in the results.[34] For example, to estimate the expected annual cost savings to plants in the proposed rule, FSIS assumed that plants participating in the optional new poultry inspection system would increase their slaughter line speeds by an average of 6 percent. However, the agency noted in a footnote in the proposed rule that line speeds could potentially increase by up to 25 percent (from 140 carcasses per minute to 175 carcasses per minute) at young chicken plants or by up to 22 percent (from 45 carcasses per minute to 55 carcasses per minute) at turkey plants. These ranges in line speed are key parameters for estimating benefits to plants and would affect the labor costs of processing each carcass, as well as the number of carcasses processed and overall profits. Although FSIS noted a range in line speed exists, it did not use a sensitivity analysis to calculate a range of annual net benefits to plants resulting from uncertainties in line speed. As a result, the public, including stakeholders, did not have complete and accurate information to inform their comments on the proposed rule and provide them with a clearer understanding of

---

[34]According to USDA's departmental regulation, it may be necessary to provide a sensitivity analysis to reveal whether, and to what extent, the results are sensitive to plausible changes in the main assumptions and numeric inputs. A sensitivity analysis is an analysis of the change in major assumptions to determine uncertainty.

the potential impacts of the final rule, including uncertainty behind selected estimates.

According to USDA's departmental regulation, uncertainty is inherent in a cost-benefit analysis, and the uncertainties that are important to regulatory decisions should be identified and presented as part of the overall regulatory analysis. According to FSIS officials, the only uncertainties that are important to this regulation are related to public health, and the agency included a range in its estimation of the public health benefits of the proposed rule. However, we believe that there are other uncertainties in the proposed rule that are important to the cost-benefit analysis, such as the expected benefit to industry from lifting the current restriction on line speed.

Third, FSIS used a variety of economic studies to assess the economic conditions in the poultry industry under the proposed rule but did not identify certain limitations of these studies, including that data in at least one of the studies were more than 20 years old. Specifically, FSIS did not disclose that these studies may not reflect current market conditions. FSIS stated that it used the best available information when it drafted the proposed rule and cited the studies in footnotes throughout the proposed rule. However, FSIS did not identify how limitations in the studies could potentially affect the overall cost-benefit analysis. For example, FSIS stated in the proposed rule that it assumed the total labor-related cost to process a bird was 15 percent on the basis of a study published in 2000, but the agency did not disclose that the study was based on data from 1972 to 1992 for chickens and from 1967 to 1992 for turkeys. As another example, FSIS estimated the mark-up price of poultry to be 10 percent more than wholesale prices based on a study published in 2000, which was based on information on the price of poultry from 1996. As a result, the public, including stakeholders, may not know if the economic conditions in the poultry industry presented in the proposed rule accurately reflect current market conditions.

According to FSIS officials, the agency plans to address some of the limitations in its revised cost-benefit analysis to support the final rule. For example, the agency plans to include a range for annual production cost savings in the revised cost-benefit analysis, which is part of the draft final rule. However, according to FSIS officials, the draft final rule is undergoing departmental review and was not made available to us, as it is subject to additional changes. It is unclear whether all of the limitations that we identified will be disclosed in the final rule.

Moreover, to estimate the public health impact of the proposed rule, FSIS developed a risk assessment that contributes to its cost-benefit analysis. FSIS' risk assessment model examined how pathogen levels in poultry products could be affected, depending on the frequency and scheduling of activities performed by FSIS inspectors positioned off the slaughter line. We were unable to determine if the results of FSIS' risk assessment accurately stated the public health benefits in the proposed rule because the risk assessment did not include sufficient detail about its methodology. According to USDA's departmental regulation and OMB Circular A-4, a good analysis is transparent, and a qualified third party reading the regulatory analysis should be able to see what data, methods, models, and assumptions were used to arrive at the agency's estimates. However, in its risk assessment, FSIS did not disclose its rationale for numerous, complex key assumptions critical to the analyses it used to calculate public health benefits for the proposed rule.[35] In addition, in the proposed rule, FSIS identified a range of 1,540 to 10,547 potential illnesses averted by increasing the number of unscheduled inspection activities off the slaughter line. However, this only covered 80 percent of the estimated range of potential illnesses averted, and it is unclear why FSIS did not disclose a wider range of potential benefits.[36] Had a wider range been used, FSIS would have increased the statistical confidence of its estimate in the number of illnesses averted by increasing unscheduled activities off the slaughter line. FSIS officials acknowledged the importance of disclosing sufficient details about the methodology and stated that the risk assessment represents a snapshot in time; they also said that a revised risk assessment supporting the final rule—an assessment that is not yet available to the public—includes more of this critical information. The revised risk assessment is part of the draft final rule that is undergoing departmental review and was not made available to us.

---

[35]For example, the basis for using certain statistical analyses (e.g., distribution of unscheduled inspection activities off the slaughter line) were not disclosed or explained.

[36]FSIS estimated that the illnesses averted would be 1,540 for the 10th percentile of the range of potential illnesses averted and 10,547 for the 90th percentile of the range of potential illnesses averted. By covering 80 percent of the possible estimated range in potential illnesses avoided, differences for results in this range could happen by chance 20 percent of the time.

Conclusions

In an effort to deploy inspection resources more effectively in accordance with food safety and other consumer protection requirements, FSIS has been conducting pilot projects at slaughter plants for young chickens, young turkeys, and young hogs since 1998. These pilot projects are in keeping with FSIS' broader effort to move toward a risk-based inspection system, which we believe is a positive step. However, we found that FSIS has not thoroughly evaluated how the three pilot projects have performed over time. Specifically, there are limitations in the agency's data analyses in its report evaluating the pilot project at young chicken plants, and there is no report evaluating the pilot project at young turkey plants. Nonetheless, the agency moved forward with a proposed rule in January 2012 on modernizing poultry slaughter inspections that included an optional new poultry inspection system, based, in part, on its experience with the pilot projects at young chicken and young turkey plants. As a result, FSIS may not have assurance that its evaluation of the pilot project at young chicken plants provides the information necessary to support the proposed rule for both chickens and turkeys. However, the agency will not complete another evaluation before it issues a final rule. To support the proposed rule, the agency developed a cost-benefit analysis but did not disclose certain limitations in sources of information—including that data in at least one study was more than 20 years old—it relied on to develop this analysis, which is not consistent with USDA regulation and OMB Circular A-4 stating that a good analysis for rulemaking is transparent. As of July 2013, FSIS officials stated that the agency plans to address some of these limitations as it works to complete the final rule. Without complete disclosure from FSIS, the public, including stakeholders, did not have complete and accurate information to inform their comments on the proposed rule and provide them with a clearer understanding of the potential impacts of the final rule, including the uncertainty behind selected estimates. By addressing these limitations moving forward in its rulemaking for modernizing poultry slaughter inspections, FSIS can prepare for more transparency in the development of a future proposed rule to modify slaughter inspection for hogs based on the pilot project at young hog plants.

In 2011, FSIS began drafting a preliminary report evaluating the pilot project at young hog plants, which uses analyses similar to those presented in the report evaluating the pilot project at young chicken plants, suggesting that similar limitations may apply. FSIS officials stated that the agency intends to complete its evaluation of the pilot project at young hog plants by March 31, 2014. They also stated that the agency would need to decide if additional data would be collected when it proceeded forward with a rulemaking effort for hogs. Without collecting and analyzing additional data, it will be difficult for FSIS to draw conclusions about whether the pilot project at young hog plants is meeting its purpose of deploying inspection resources more effectively in accordance with food safety and other consumer protection requirements. Because the pilot project at young hog plants is ongoing, FSIS has the opportunity to follow sound management practices by planning for and collecting key information needed to determine whether the pilot project is meeting its purpose. As we have previously reported, pilot programs can more effectively inform future program rollout when sound management practices are followed.

Recommendations for Executive Action

We recommend that the Secretary of Agriculture direct the Administrator of the Food Safety and Inspection Service to take the following two actions:

- Clearly disclose to the public limitations in the information—including the cost-benefit analysis—the agency relied on for the rulemaking to modernize poultry slaughter inspections.
- As FSIS continues its evaluation of its pilot project for young hogs, collect and analyze the information necessary to determine whether the pilot project is meeting its purpose.

Agency Comments and Our Evaluation

We provided a draft of this report to USDA for its review and comment. USDA's written comments and our detailed response to them are reproduced in appendix III. In its written comments, USDA concurred with both of our recommendations. More specifically, USDA concurred with our recommendation that it clearly disclose to the public limitations in the information—including the cost-benefit analysis—it relied on for the rulemaking to modernize poultry slaughter inspections. According to USDA, when it issues the final rule, it will present the updated analyses in a manner that will facilitate the public's understanding of the information used to support its rulemaking. USDA also concurred with our recommendation to collect and analyze the information necessary to determine whether the pilot project for young hogs is meeting its purpose, while continuing its evaluation of this pilot project. According to USDA, it plans to complete such an evaluation by March 31, 2014, at which time it will determine whether a permanent program is warranted.

USDA also made several general comments. For example, USDA commented that, throughout our report, we state that the purpose of the pilot projects was to "…deploy inspection resources more effectively…".

USDA further commented that, while this might have been true when the pilot projects were initiated in 1997, the agency's thinking has evolved over the years to focus less on efficiencies and more on public health and food safety. We recognize that USDA's descriptions of the pilot projects, as stated in the *Federal Register* notices, have evolved over the years. However, we believe that the purpose stated in our report—deploying inspection resources more effectively in accordance with food safety and other consumer protection requirements—remains valid because the *Federal Register* notices cited by USDA continue to mention effective use of resources as a component of its pilot projects. Moreover, agency officials directed us to the *Federal Register* notices because the agency could not provide us with documents defining the pilot projects' purpose. As our report states, pilot programs can more effectively inform future program rollout when sound management practices are followed, including the development of an evaluation plan with well-defined, clear, and measurable objectives.

Furthermore, USDA provided technical comments in its written response, which we have incorporated, as appropriate, in the report.

As agreed with your office, unless you publicly announce the contents of this report earlier, we plan no further distribution until 30 days from the report date. At that time, we will send copies of this report to the Secretary of Agriculture, the appropriate congressional committees, and other interested parties. In addition, the report will be available at no charge on the GAO website at http://www.gao.gov.

If you or your staff members have any questions regarding this report, please contact me at (202) 512-3841 or gomezj@gao.gov. Contact points for our Offices of Congressional Relations and Public Affairs may be found on the last page of this report. Key contributors to this report are listed in appendix IV.

Sincerely yours,

J. Alfredo Gómez
Director, Natural Resources and Environment

Appendix I: Objectives, Scope, and Methodology

This report responds to your request that we review U.S. Department of Agriculture's (USDA) pilot projects at slaughter plants for young chickens, young turkeys, and young hogs. Our objectives were to determine (1) the extent to which USDA has evaluated the three pilot projects, (2) strengths and weaknesses of the three pilot projects based on the views of key stakeholder groups, and (3) the extent to which USDA disclosed limitations, if any, in sources of information it relied on to develop the proposed rule to modernize poultry slaughter inspections.

To determine the extent to which USDA has evaluated the three pilot projects, we reviewed relevant USDA documents, *Federal Register* notices, and laws. We also compared USDA's efforts to evaluate the pilot projects with criteria based on social science and evaluation literature and published GAO guidance that were identified in our previous work on pilot program development and evaluation. Our previous work dealt with pilot projects at the Federal Emergency Management Agency, the Internal Revenue Service, and the Department of Defense where we identified key features of a well-developed evaluation plan that increases the likelihood that evaluations would yield methodologically sound results and support effective program and policy decisions.[1] We believe that the key features identified in those reports are applicable to pilot projects, in general, including USDA's three pilot projects. In addition, we interviewed several officials in various offices within USDA's Food Safety and Inspection Service—the agency responsible for USDA's meat and poultry inspection program.

To determine the strengths and weaknesses of the three pilot projects based on the views of key stakeholder groups, we identified key stakeholder groups representing industry, labor (including plant personnel and USDA inspectors and veterinarians), consumer advocacy, and animal welfare that submitted comments on USDA's proposed rule on

---

[1] GAO-11-383, GAO-09-45, and GAO-06-538. Specifically, in GAO-11-383, GAO-09-45, and GAO-06-538, we reported that a sound, well-developed and documented evaluation plan includes, at a minimum: (1) well-defined, clear, and measurable objectives; (2) criteria or standards for determining pilot-program performance; (3) clearly articulated methodology, including sound sampling methods, determination of appropriate sample size for the evaluation design, and a strategy for comparing the pilot results with other efforts; (4) a clear plan that details the type and source of data necessary to evaluate the pilot, methods for data collection, and the timing and frequency of data collection; and (5) a data analysis plan to track the program's performance and evaluate the final results of the project.

modernizing poultry slaughter inspections. We identified 11 key
stakeholder groups with sufficient knowledge about USDA's pilot projects
at young chicken, young turkey, and young hog plants to identify
strengths and weaknesses for these pilot projects.[2] These stakeholder
groups were the American Federation of Government
Employees/National Joint Council of Food Inspection Locals, the
American Meat Institute, the Center for Foodborne Illness Research and
Prevention, the Consumer Federation of America, Food and Water
Watch, the Government Accountability Project, the Humane Society of
the United States, the National Association of Federal Veterinarians, the
National Chicken Council, the National Turkey Federation, and the North
American Meat Association.[3] We reviewed their comments to USDA's
proposed rule to determine the extent to which the comments may apply
to the pilot projects; interviewed representatives of these key stakeholder
groups; and followed up with e-mailed questions to gauge their level of
familiarity with each pilot project and then clarified responses, as needed.
Three of our analysts worked together to develop categories of strengths
and weaknesses identified most frequently by stakeholder groups, and
two analysts independently determined whether each stakeholder group
had identified strengths or weaknesses that fit into these categories. Any
discrepancies in coding were discussed, and agreement was reached
between the analysts, or resolved through a third analyst's review. We
also visited 10 slaughter plants for young chickens, young turkeys, and
young hogs to learn about the variations in slaughter inspection systems
between plants participating and not participating in the pilot projects. In
selecting these plants, we chose plants in states that are the top
producers of young chickens, young turkeys, and young hogs and that
have at least one plant that is participating in a pilot project and at least
one plant that is not participating in a pilot project for one of those
species. On the basis of these selection criteria, we visited plants in
Georgia for young chickens, Indiana for young turkeys, and Minnesota for

[2]We developed an initial list of key stakeholder groups based on our prior experience and
knowledge. To ensure that we included all of the relevant stakeholder groups, we asked
these groups for suggestions on other stakeholders we should consider contacting and
expanded the list, as needed.

[3]The Center for Science in the Public Interest was also included in our methodology but
we were unsuccessful in obtaining an interview. We also contacted People for the Ethical
Treatment of Animals and the United Food and Commercial Workers International Union,
but these stakeholder groups did not respond to our e-mail questions specific to strengths
and weaknesses of USDA's pilot projects.

GAO-13-775 USDA Inspection Pilot Projects

young hogs. For each species, we visited at least one plant participating and one plant not participating in the pilot projects. We interviewed plant management and USDA veterinarians and inspectors working at these plants, and we toured the plants.

To determine the extent to which USDA disclosed limitations, if any, in sources of information it relied on to develop the proposed rule, we reviewed the proposed rule and related *Federal Register* notices, as well as selected documents the agency relied on to develop the proposed rule. We also reviewed relevant guidance such as the Office of Management and Budget Circular A-4,[4] which provides guidance to federal agencies on the development of regulatory analysis, and the USDA departmental regulation that details the process for developing regulations.[5] We also interviewed several officials in various offices within USDA's Food Safety and Inspection Service to clarify information, as needed.

We conducted this performance audit from September 2012 to August 2013 in accordance with generally accepted government auditing standards. Those standards require that we plan and perform the audit to obtain sufficient, appropriate evidence to provide a reasonable basis for our findings and conclusions based on our audit objectives. We believe that the evidence presented provides a reasonable basis for our findings and conclusions based on our audit objectives.

---

[4]OMB, Circular A-4, Sept. 17, 2003.

[5]USDA, Departmental Regulation, No. 1512, Regulatory Decision Making Requirements, Dec. 24, 2008.

Appendix II: Additional Information on the Young Chicken, Young Turkey, and Young Hog Plants in the Pilot Projects

As of July 2013, 29 plants were participating in the pilot projects in 18 states. More specifically, there were 19 participating young chicken plants located in 10 states. These 10 states accounted for almost 66 percent of the more than 49.3 billion pounds of young chickens slaughtered in 2012.[1] (See fig. 2.)

---

[1]We used 2012 data on the annual volume of chickens slaughtered, by state, because those are the most recent data available. The states with plants that were participating in the pilot project, as of July 2013, were the same states as in 2012. In 2011, one plant dropped out of the pilot project for young chickens and closed its operations. If this plant is included, then the 20 young chicken plants in the pilot project were located in 11 states. Because this plant closed its operations in 2011, it did not contribute to the total volume of young chickens slaughtered in 2012.

Appendix II: Additional Information on the
Young Chicken, Young Turkey, and Young Hog
Plants in the Pilot Projects

Figure 2: Location of Young Chicken Plants in the Pilot Project and the Volume of Young Chickens Slaughtered, by State, in 2012

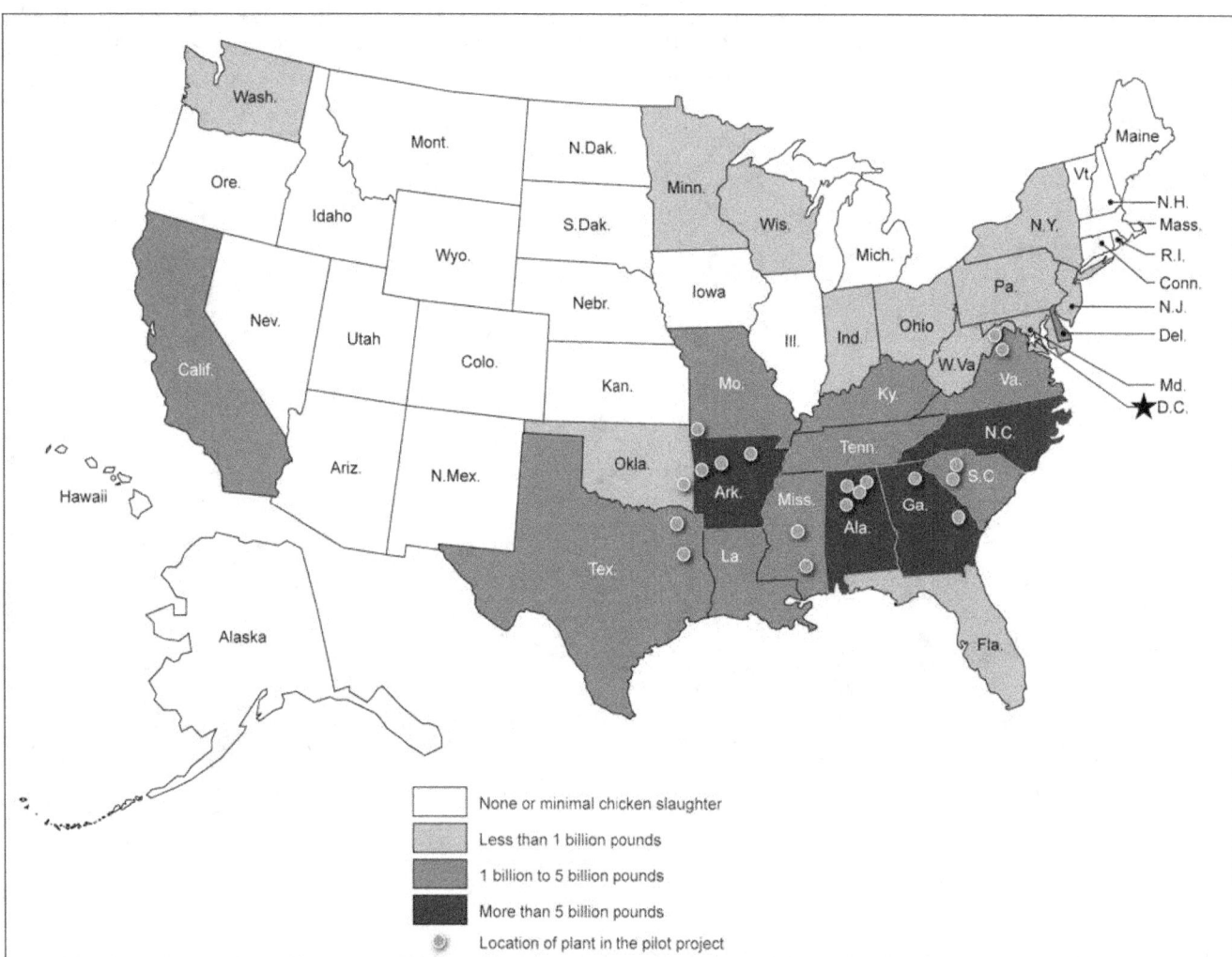

Sources: GAO presentation of U.S. Department of Agriculture information; Map Resources (map).

Note: Information on volumes was for the total live weight of young chickens slaughtered. According to USDA, the agency did not publish all of the data by individual states to avoid disclosure in states with low slaughter volumes. These states were included in the "None or minimal slaughter" category and collectively slaughtered about 140 million pounds of young chickens. In 2012, in the 26 states where young chickens were slaughtered and for which data were reported, the volumes slaughtered ranged from about 8.2 million to almost 6.8 billion pounds per state.

Appendix II: Additional Information on the
Young Chicken, Young Turkey, and Young Hog
Plants in the Pilot Projects

In terms of the pilot project at young turkey plants, four of the five young turkey plants in the pilot project were located in states that accounted for about 33 percent of the more than 7.4 billion pounds of young turkeys slaughtered in 2012; one young turkey plant was located in Michigan—a state with a lower volume of young turkeys slaughtered—and data were not available on the volume of young turkeys slaughtered in this state.[2] (See fig. 3.)

---

[2]We used 2012 data on the annual volume of turkeys slaughtered, by state, because those are the most recent data available. The states with plants that were participating in the pilot project, as of July 2013, were the same states as in 2012.

Appendix II: Additional Information on the
Young Chicken, Young Turkey, and Young Hog
Plants in the Pilot Projects

Figure 3: Location of Young Turkey Plants in the Pilot Project and the Volume of Young Turkeys Slaughtered, by State, in 2012

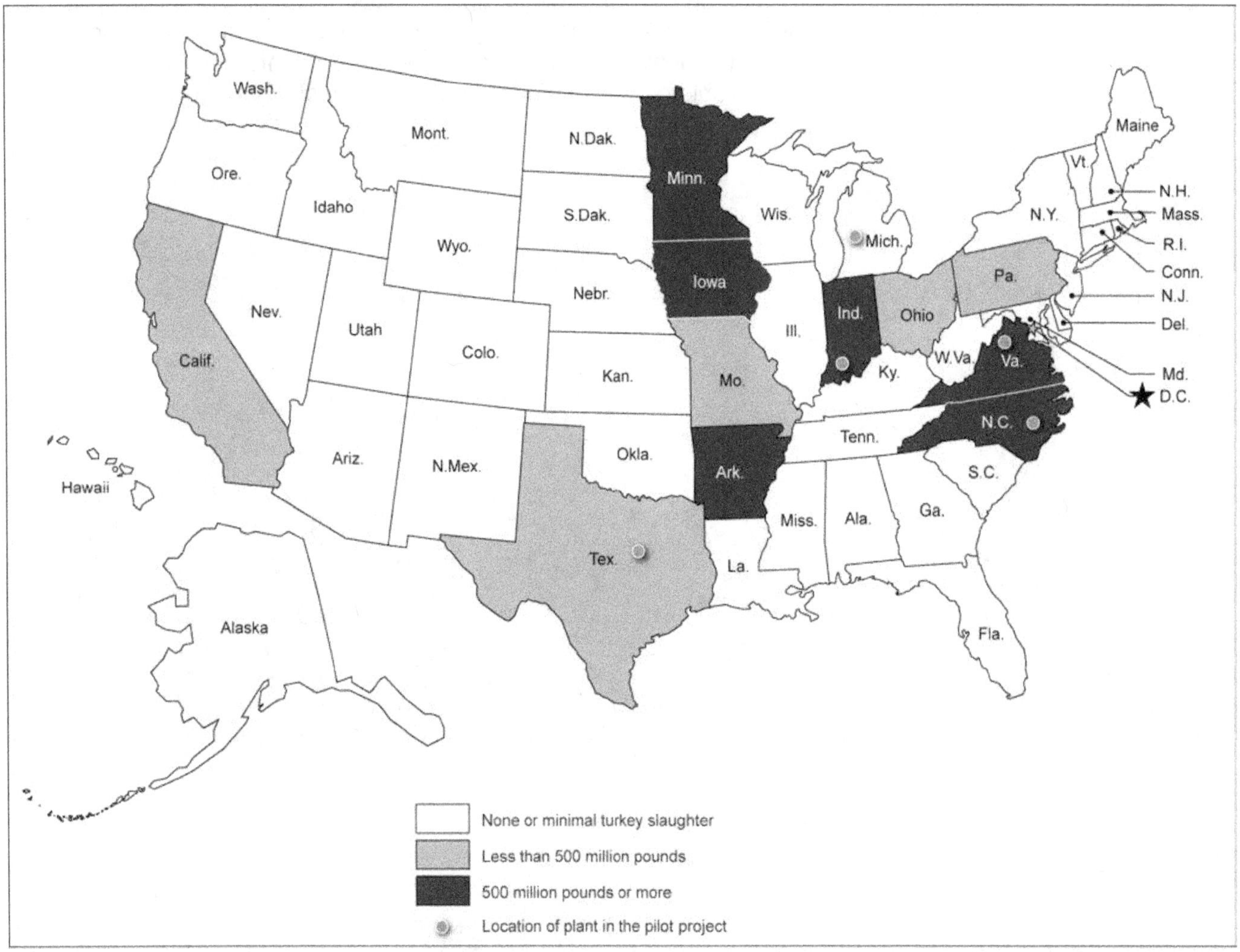

Sources: GAO presentation of U.S. Department of Agriculture information; Map Resources (map).

Note: Information on volumes was for the total live weight of young turkeys slaughtered. According to USDA, the agency did not publish all of the data by individual states to avoid disclosure in states with low slaughter volumes. These states were included in the "None or minimal slaughter" category and collectively slaughtered about 1.2 billion pounds of young turkeys. In 2012, in the 11 states where young turkeys were slaughtered and for which data were reported, the volumes slaughtered ranged from about 111 million pounds to more than 1.1 billion pounds per state.

**Appendix II: Additional Information on the
Young Chicken, Young Turkey, and Young Hog
Plants in the Pilot Projects**

In terms of the pilot project at young hog plants, the five hog plants in the pilot project were located in five states that accounted for about 30 percent of the more than 31 billion pounds of hogs slaughtered in 2012.[3] (See fig. 4.)

---

[3]We used 2012 data on the annual volume of hogs slaughtered, by state, because those are the most recent data available. The states with plants that were participating in the pilot project, as of July 2013, were the same states as in 2012.

Appendix II: Additional Information on the
Young Chicken, Young Turkey, and Young Hog
Plants in the Pilot Projects

Figure 4: Location of Young Hog Plants in the Pilot Project and the Volume of Hogs Slaughtered, by State, in 2012

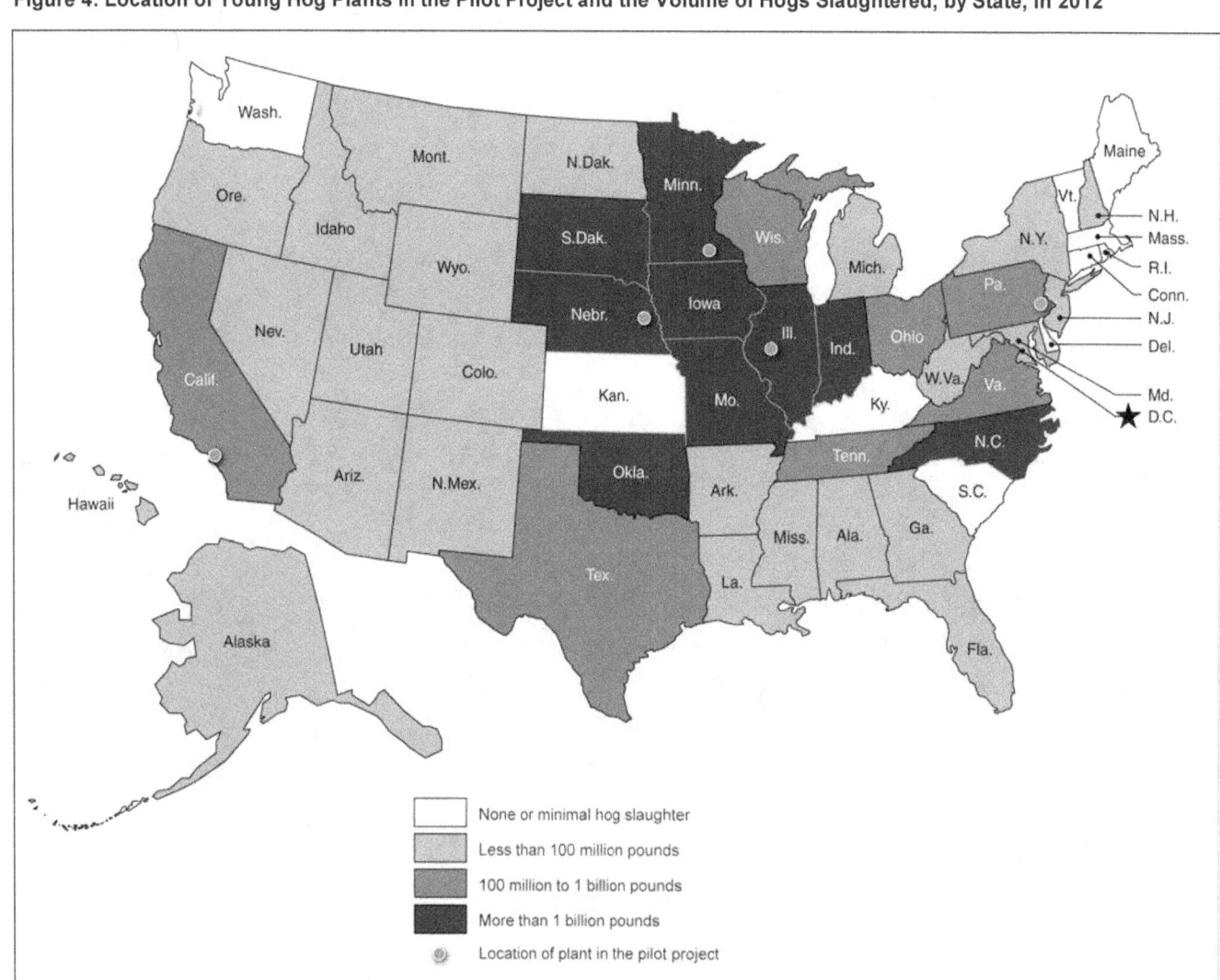

Legend:
- None or minimal hog slaughter
- Less than 100 million pounds
- 100 million to 1 billion pounds
- More than 1 billion pounds
- Location of plant in the pilot project

Sources: GAO presentation of U.S. Department of Agriculture information; Map Resources (map).

Note: Information on volumes was for the total live weight of hogs slaughtered commercially, which includes hogs slaughtered in federally inspected plants and other plants but excludes animals slaughtered on farms. USDA's slaughter statistics did not distinguish between young and mature hogs. According to USDA, the agency did not publish all of the data by individual states to avoid disclosure in states with low slaughter volumes. These states were included in the "None or minimal slaughter" category and collectively slaughtered about 1 billion pounds of young hogs. The volume for Maryland included the slaughter information from Delaware, and the volume for New Hampshire included the slaughter information from other New England states—Connecticut, Maine, Massachusetts, Rhode Island, and Vermont. In 2012, in the 40 states where hogs were slaughtered and for which data were reported, the volumes slaughtered ranged from about 151,000 pounds to over 8.2 billion pounds per state.

Appendix III: Comments from the U.S. Department of Agriculture

Note: GAO comments supplementing those in the report text appear at the end of this appendix.

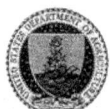

DEPARTMENT OF AGRICULTURE

OFFICE OF THE SECRETARY

WASHINGTON, D.C. 20250

AUG 1 5 2013

J. Alfredo Gómez
Director
Natural Resources and Environment
United States Government Accountability Office
441 G. Street, N.W.
Washington, D.C., 20508

Dear Mr. Gómez,

The United States Department of Agriculture (USDA) appreciates the opportunity to review the U.S. Government Accountability Office's (GAO) draft report entitled *Food Safety: More Disclosure and Data Needed to Clarify Impact of Changes to Poultry and Hog Inspections* (GAO-13-775). USDA appreciates GAO's work in planning, conducting and issuing this report.

See comment 1.

We would like to make a few general comments. While the GAO report highlights some of the objectives of the Proposed Poultry Slaughter Rule (PSR), it does not highlight what FSIS considers the main objectives of this rule. GAO has emphasized the need to reduce overlap of food safety duties "...to ensure the effective use of scarce government resources."[1] The PSR will reduce overlap of duties between plant employees and FSIS inspection program personnel (IPP) by focusing IPP on areas of greatest risk. As stated by Secretary Vilsack, "The new inspection system will reduce the risk of foodborne illness by focusing FSIS inspection activities on those tasks that advance our core mission of food safety. By revising current procedures and removing outdated regulatory requirements that do not help combat foodborne illness, the result will be a more efficient and effective use of taxpayer dollars." In addition, the proposed requirements which will apply to all plants that slaughter poultry, except for ratites, represent significant advances over the pilot project and current poultry slaughter inspection. For example, the proposed requirements will require poultry slaughter plants to develop written procedures to prevent contamination of carcasses and parts that must include, at a minimum, sampling and analysis for microbial organisms at the pre-chill and post-chill points in the process to monitor process control for enteric pathogens.

See comment 2.

We also noted that, throughout this report, GAO states that the purpose of HIMP was to "...deploy inspection resources more effectively...." While this might have been

---

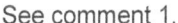

[1] GAO, *Oversight of Food Safety Activities: Federal Agencies Should Pursue Opportunities to Reduce Overlap and Better Leverage Resources*, GAO-05-213 (Washington, D.C.: March 2005)

J. Alfredo Gómez
Page 2

true when the HIMP project was initiated in July 10, 1997, FSIS' thinking with respect to HIMP has evolved over the years to focus less on efficiencies and more on public health and food safety. In an FR Notice dated July 29, 1998 (Volume 63, Number 145)], FSIS states that "[t]he HACCP-Based Inspection Models project is intended to produce a more flexible, efficient, and fully integrated system of oversight and controls. FSIS expects this system of establishment controls and Agency oversight and verification to yield increased food-safety and other benefits to consumers." In November 2, 2000, FSIS issued another FR Notice (Volume 65, Number 213) which states that "FSIS began HIMP in 1998 to determine whether new government slaughter inspection procedures, along with new plant responsibilities, can improve food safety and increase consumer protection." This evolution is also mentioned in an FR Notice dated July 31, 2007 (Volume 72, Number 146) which states "[t]he Agency's thinking has evolved and benefited from its experience with the Hazard Analysis and Critical Control Point (HACCP)-based Inspection Models Project (HIMP). The new system will be designed to provide more time and more flexibility than the current systems for FSIS personnel to conduct focused, off-line verification activities according to risk factors at each establishment and at points in slaughter and processing where food safety hazards and associated risks may be introduced." Further, in FSIS' report, *Evaluation of HACCP Inspection Models Project (HIMP)*, dated August 2011, the purpose of the evaluation was not to determine whether inspection efficiencies were realized but "....to determine whether the HIMP inspection system results in improved safety of poultry products and increased overall consumer protection, while ensuring carcass-by-carcass inspection of each eviscerated carcass." Based on the results of our evaluation, FSIS determined that an inspection system based on the HIMP system "... will ensure an equivalent, if not better, level of food safety and other consumer protection than that provided by the existing poultry slaughter inspection systems."

See comment 3.

We would also like to note that the external review[2] found that FSIS' approach for comparing food quality data, and more importantly, its approach for comparing food safety data, is valid and supported the HIMP study design. While the GAO draft report indicates that the approach for comparing food quality data is valid, the GAO draft report fails to mention that the review found FSIS' approach for comparing food safety data valid as well. In addition, the GAO draft report also fails to include a number of the conclusions from the external review that supported the HIMP study design.

See comment 4.

FSIS would also like to clarify and correct statements made in the report. On page 7 related to the discussion of performance standards, the report states that "FSIS set performance standards for food safety defects at zero...," and footnote 11 states that "[t]he Agency developed the performance standard of zero to allow it to compare performance between plants participating and not participating in the pilot projects."

---

[2] B.M. Hargis, P.A. Curtis, M.G. Johnson and J.D. Williams, *Review of the HACCP-Based Inspection Models Project by the National Alliance for Food Safety Technical Team,* (2002)

J. Alfredo Gómez
Page 3

This is not quite accurate. The Agency has a zero tolerance for food safety defects, i.e. septicemia/toxemia and visible fecal, in both HIMP and non-HIMP plants. On page 22 of FSIS' August 2011 report, *Evaluation of the HACCP Inspection Models Project (HIMP)*, it explains that, for comparison purposes, FSIS developed food safety performance standards for septicemia/toxemia and visible fecal set at the 75th percentile of what was achieved under the RTI baseline study. The HIMP report compares young chicken HIMP plants' performance with the HIMP food safety performance standards.

See comment 5.

On page 14, the report states that "….the agency analyzed the relationship between the frequency with which FSIS inspectors positioned off the slaughter line at five young turkey plants…." FSIS would like to emphasize that the Agency analyzed the relationship between pathogen presence/absence and the frequency with which FSIS inspectors carried out specific off-line inspection activities in more than just five young turkey establishments. Specifically, FSIS did evaluate inspection data and *Salmonella* and *Campylobacter* data from turkey slaughter establishments in the conduct of its peer reviewed quantitative microbial risk assessment. This risk assessment was based on available paired data for *Salmonella* occurrence data in **65** turkey establishments. Similarly *Campylobacter* data represented **58** turkey establishments. This data represented more than 90% of turkey slaughter annually.

See comment 6.

On page 20 of the report in which training is discussed, it states that "[a]ccording to FSIS officials, training of plant personnel was not required or necessary because…" We did not say that training was not necessary. In the proposed rule, we said that proper training of plant employees was important to plant sorter's ability to make accurate decisions, and that if sorters do not make appropriate decisions, inspectors will be required to take actions such as stopping the line, issuing NRs, and directing plants to reduce line speeds. (77 FR 4419.) Thus, establishments will have a significant incentive to properly train their employees. We also said that under the proposed rule, establishments would have the flexibility to select the training program that will best assist them to meet the requirements of the proposed rule, and that we would issue compliance guidance for how to train establishment sorters.

See comment 7.

The second bullet point on page 22 includes the following statement: "More specifically, the FSIS inspector positioned on the line could no longer cite the plant for non-compliances with FSIS' zero tolerance standard for visible fecal material, because the plant would not yet have an opportunity to control this hazard." This statement is misleading because it implies that FSIS online inspectors in non-HIMP plants currently issue NRs for non-compliance with the zero tolerance for visible fecal material. This is not the case. Online inspectors in non-HIMP plants do not issue NRs if they observe visible fecal material. Carcasses with visible fecal are permitted to proceed down the line and be re-processed to remove the visible fecal. There is no additional online inspection after the plant reprocesses carcasses to verify that the visible fecal contamination has been removed.

J. Alfredo Gómez
Page 4

GAO states on page 25 of its report that "FSIS did not include a sensitivity analysis or range for the potential increase in line speed, which would affect the labor costs of processing each carcass as well as the number of carcasses processed and overall process," even though it acknowledges earlier in the paragraph that "the agency noted in a footnote to the proposed rule that line speeds could potentially increase by up to 25 percent . . . at young chicken plants or by up to 22 percent . . .at young turkey plants." It should state "at turkey plants," not "young" turkey plants. In addition, the paragraph is misleading because it implies that FSIS did not present a range for the line speed, which it did, in the footnote, as indicated in the report. It is also misleading because it implies that a higher line speed than the average used in the analysis, would lead to additional costs of processing that were not mentioned in the analysis. The FSIS treatment of these costs was to offset them against the reduced costs per bird from the increased line speed. Therefore, any increase in line speed above the average used in the analysis (6 %) would result in a net reduction in per unit costs for processing birds to these establishments, which will result in higher benefits. This description is spelled out in the proposed rule and makes the treatment of line speed costs and benefits transparent to the public.

On page 26 of the report, GAO states that: "the agency plans to address some of these limitations in its cost-benefit analysis to support the final rule, including a range for annual production cost savings to industry, based on a range of line speeds." This is not completely accurate. The following clarifies how we plan to address some of the limitations in the cost-benefit analysis:

- The draft Final Regulatory Impact Analysis (FRIA) now has a range for annual production cost savings. The Proposed Regulatory Impact Analysis (PRIA) did not provide a range for annual cost savings.
- The draft FRIA does not provide a range for the 6 percent since this number is supported by the HIMP pilot project data. The resulting annual production savings are presented with a range, though, in the draft FRIA, as mentioned in the previous bullet.

We would also suggest deleting in the second full paragraph on page 26 the phrase "....based on a range of line speeds."

On pages 26-27, GAO discusses the limitations of the risk assessment; however, FSIS has revised this risk assessment, and it now addresses these limitations. The last paragraph before the conclusion accurately summarizes the conversation that FSIS had with GAO concerning updates to the risk assessment that were unavailable to GAO but will be part of the final rule.

Recommendation 1:
Clearly disclose to the public limitations in the information—including the cost-benefit analysis—the agency relied on for the rulemaking to modernize poultry slaughter inspections.

See comment 8.

See comment 9.

J. Alfredo Gómez
Page 5

<u>USDA Response:</u>
FSIS concurs with this recommendation. FSIS has updated the analyses used to
support the proposed rule, and the results continue to support moving forward with a
final rule to modernize poultry slaughter inspection. When it issues the final rule,
FSIS will present the updated analyses, including the cost-benefit analysis, in a
manner that will facilitate public understanding of the information used to support the
rulemaking.

<u>Recommendation 2:</u>
As USDA continues its evaluation of its pilot project for [market] hogs, collect and
analyze the information necessary to determine whether the pilot project is meeting
its purpose.

<u>USDA Response:</u>
FSIS concurs with this recommendation. FSIS will complete an evaluation of HIMP
market hog establishments to determine whether the pilot project is meeting its
purpose. The report will include an analysis of market hog HIMP establishments'
performance compared to non-HIMP market hog establishments as well as their
performance with respect to performance standards established by an independent
consulting firm contractor. Such an evaluation may support rule-making to amend
regulations to make an inspection system informed by the market hog HIMP pilot
permanent. FSIS will complete this evaluation and determine if a permanent program
is warranted by March 31, 2014.

Again, thank you for the opportunity to review and comment on this draft report. We
look forward to working with you on future Department of Agriculture engagements.

Sincerely,

Elisabeth A. Hagen, M.D.
Under Secretary
Food Safety

GAO Comments

The following are GAO's comments on the U.S. Department of Agriculture's letter dated August 15, 2013.

1. USDA commented that our report does not highlight what the agency considers to be the main objectives of the proposed rule to modernize poultry slaughter inspections—to reduce the risk of foodborne illnesses by focusing FSIS inspection activities on those tasks that advance the agency's core mission of food safety. However, our report includes this information. For example, our report states, "according to the proposed rule, the modernization is intended to improve food safety and the effectiveness of poultry slaughter inspection systems, remove unnecessary regulatory obstacles to innovation, and make better use of the agency's resources," among other things.

2. USDA commented that throughout our report we state that the purpose of the pilot projects was to "...deploy inspection resources more effectively...". USDA further commented that, while this might have been true when the pilot projects were initiated in 1997, the agency's thinking has evolved over the years to focus less on efficiencies and more on public health and food safety. We recognize that USDA's descriptions of the pilot projects, as stated in the *Federal Register* notices, have evolved over the years. However, we believe that the purpose stated in our report—deploying inspection resources more effectively in accordance with food safety and other consumer protection requirements—remains valid because the *Federal Register* notices cited by USDA continue to mention the effective use of resources as a component of its pilot projects. Moreover, agency officials directed us to *Federal Register* notices because USDA could not provide us with documents defining the pilot projects' purpose. As our report states, pilot programs can more effectively inform future program rollout when sound management practices are followed, including the development of an evaluation plan with well-defined, clear, and measurable objectives.

3. USDA commented that we did not mention the validity of the agency's approach for comparing food safety data. We modified our report to include this information. USDA also commented that we did not include a number of conclusions from a 2002 external review, which focused on the validity of using food safety, microbial, and other consumer protection (food quality) data to assess the accomplishments of young chicken plants participating in and those not participating in the pilot project. Our report acknowledges this external review, but looking at the validity of the performance measures the agency developed for the pilot project was beyond the scope of our review.

4. We modified our report to clarify the footnote about the food safety performance standard.

5. We modified our report to clarify the description of how the data from young turkey plants were used in USDA's risk assessment.

6. We modified our report to clarify USDA's perspective on training and that this training discussion is specific to those plants participating in the pilot projects.

7. We modified our report to include a statement about USDA inspectors' abilities to cite plants for noncompliance at plants not participating in the pilot project.

8. USDA commented that our discussion of line speed is misleading because, among other things, it implies that a higher line speed than the average used in the analysis would lead to additional costs of processing. We recognize that higher line speeds lead to lower per unit labor costs and have not made statements to the contrary. However, we note that USDA did not incorporate the impact of a range in line speeds in its estimates of benefits to plants. These ranges in line speed are key parameters for estimating benefits to plants and would affect the labor costs of processing each carcass, as well as the number of carcasses processed and overall profits. We modified our report to clarify that although FSIS noted a range in line speed exists, it did not use a sensitivity analysis to calculate a range of annual net benefits to plants resulting from uncertainties in line speed.

9. USDA commented that our statement about how the agency plans to address some of the limitations in the cost-benefit analysis is not completely accurate. We modified our report to state that the agency plans to include a range for annual production cost savings in the revised cost-benefit analysis, which is part of the draft final rule. However, USDA also stated that the final rule will not provide a range of benefits to plants based on uncertainties in line speed. As explained above in comment 8, we believe line speed is a key parameter in the estimation of benefits to plants.

Appendix IV: GAO Contact and Staff Acknowledgments

GAO Contact	J. Alfredo Gómez, (202) 512-3841 or gomezj@gao.gov.
Staff Acknowledgments	In addition to the contact named above, Mary Denigan-Macauley (Assistant Director), Marie Bancroft, Kevin Bray, Stephen Carter, Barbara El Osta, Michele Fejfar, Diana C. Goody, Armetha Liles, Cynthia Norris, and Dae Park made key contributions to this report.

GAO's Mission	The Government Accountability Office, the audit, evaluation, and investigative arm of Congress, exists to support Congress in meeting its constitutional responsibilities and to help improve the performance and accountability of the federal government for the American people. GAO examines the use of public funds; evaluates federal programs and policies; and provides analyses, recommendations, and other assistance to help Congress make informed oversight, policy, and funding decisions. GAO's commitment to good government is reflected in its core values of accountability, integrity, and reliability.
Obtaining Copies of GAO Reports and Testimony	The fastest and easiest way to obtain copies of GAO documents at no cost is through GAO's website (http://www.gao.gov). Each weekday afternoon, GAO posts on its website newly released reports, testimony, and correspondence. To have GAO e-mail you a list of newly posted products, go to http://www.gao.gov and select "E-mail Updates."
Order by Phone	The price of each GAO publication reflects GAO's actual cost of production and distribution and depends on the number of pages in the publication and whether the publication is printed in color or black and white. Pricing and ordering information is posted on GAO's website, http://www.gao.gov/ordering.htm. Place orders by calling (202) 512-6000, toll free (866) 801-7077, or TDD (202) 512-2537. Orders may be paid for using American Express, Discover Card, MasterCard, Visa, check, or money order. Call for additional information.
Connect with GAO	Connect with GAO on Facebook, Flickr, Twitter, and YouTube. Subscribe to our RSS Feeds or E-mail Updates. Listen to our Podcasts. Visit GAO on the web at www.gao.gov.
To Report Fraud, Waste, and Abuse in Federal Programs	Contact: Website: http://www.gao.gov/fraudnet/fraudnet.htm E-mail: fraudnet@gao.gov Automated answering system: (800) 424-5454 or (202) 512-7470
Congressional Relations	Katherine Siggerud, Managing Director, siggerudk@gao.gov, (202) 512-4400, U.S. Government Accountability Office, 441 G Street NW, Room 7125, Washington, DC 20548
Public Affairs	Chuck Young, Managing Director, youngc1@gao.gov, (202) 512-4800 U.S. Government Accountability Office, 441 G Street NW, Room 7149 Washington, DC 20548

Please Print on Recycled Paper.